THE EASY
KETO
INSTANT POT
COOKBOOK

150

**Delicious and Tested High-fat, Low-carb
Recipes for Losing Weight and Living Healthy**

Jamie Michael

Content

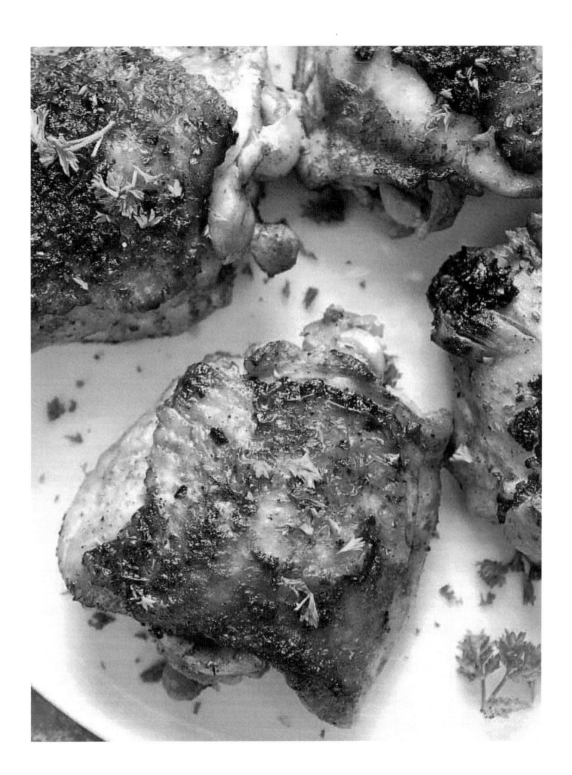

Introduction

Three years ago, I was obese. I weighed 230 pounds, and my medical bill was a testament to how unhealthy I was at that weight. After the fifth visit in a matter of months, my doctor said the only way to get healthy was to drop 50 pounds. He had in the past recommended that I go on a diet, but this time, there was more urgency in his voice.

I was at a tipping point; either lose weight or become one of the 34.2 million Americans who have diabetes (Centers for Disease Control and Prevention, 2020). My doctor suggested I try the ketogenic diet. He explained how a diet high in carbohydrates might be the reason behind my weight gain, feeling tired all the time, the constant headaches, and, of course, the high blood sugar levels (Kroemer et al., 2018).

After doing some research and consulting a dietician, I decided that a low-carb, high-fat diet would be my ticket to better health. And I haven't looked back.

Not only have I lost the 50 pounds, but my cholesterol is also looking great, I don't experience blood sugar spikes anymore, and I'm more energetic and happier overall.

I'm not going to lie; it was challenging to transition to eat the keto way. When you first start, your body goes through the process of switching its fuel source. Where carbohydrates were your body's primary energy source, it now has to adapt to using fat. You can imagine that this can be quite a shock on the body, so you may experience the keto flu in the beginning. Luckily, if you stick to the keto diet and fight any temptation to sneak in a slice of bread or other starchy food, the switch from carbs to fat happens fast.

Before changing my diet, I used my Instant Pot daily. One of my worries was that I would be forced to spend hours in the kitchen preparing keto-friendly meals, and my Instant Pot would become a white elephant. If that were to happen, I just knew I wouldn't stick to the keto diet. I work from nine to five and just don't have the time (or the inspiration) to cook after a busy day.

Well, I am happy to tell you that the keto diet is Instant-Pot friendly.

In this book, I will share with you how to get healthy without having to waste endless hours preparing food. I want to make weight loss easy for you because I've been where you are and want you to experience how it feels when your whole life doesn't revolve around your next starchy meal. Did you know that eating a lot of carbohydrates makes you eat more (Roberts, 2000)? You're always craving more and more, and in the end, all you're left with is an ever-expanding waistline and a high medical bill.

Let's get started. I can't wait to pack as much information into these pages so that you will feel confident enough to not only start the ketogenic diet but also use your Instant Pot to prepare these low-carb, high-fat meals.

CHAPTER 1
What is
the Ketogenic Diet

The ketogenic (keto for short) diet is one of the most popular ways of eating to not only lose weight but get healthy. With mounting evidence that the keto diet protects against brain disorders such as Parkinson's, Alzheimer's, and autism, the weight loss ends up looking pretty inconsequential (Campos, 2017). But considering all the negative health issues that come with being obese, keto ends up being a powerful player in maintaining overall health.

The keto diet limits the number of carbohydrates you may eat, while increasing how much fat and protein you consume. The low carb intake switches your body from using the glucose that you get from eating carbs as fuel to using ketones. Your liver produces ketones from fat—this means all the excess fat stores on your body end up being used as energy. This metabolic state is called ketosis.

Not only is it great for weight loss, but your body will also have a constant source of energy, which means fewer hunger pangs throughout the day and increased energy. Also, your body's blood sugar levels will be more stable because it won't go through the daily roller coaster of insulin spikes and blood sugar drops associated with eating starchy meals.

How Do Ketones Work?

I mentioned ketones and ketosis earlier on in this book, but I think it is good for you to know how this process works so that you're aware of what to expect.

Before starting a low-carb diet, your body runs on glucose metabolism. This means every time after eating, your blood glucose spikes, which causes more insulin to be released. This roller coaster your blood sugar and insulin levels go through is bad for your health. It promotes the storage of body fat and even blocks the use of your fat stores. Never mind that excess glucose can lead to insulin resistance and eventually lead to type 2 diabetes.

However, when there isn't enough insulin in your body to turn the glucose you get from carbohydrates into energy, your liver produces ketones. Since your body needs energy and there aren't any glucose stores to use, it is forced to go to plan B—ketones. As soon as your body completely relies on ketones as an energy source, then you enter a metabolic state called ketosis. This usually takes around two weeks, depending on your muscles' glucose stores, as well as how much you cut your carb intake. If you have 0.5 mmol/L or higher ketones in your blood, then you are in ketosis.

Your body will then be used to utilizing your fat stores and any fat that you eat for fuel. It won't be very efficient at it in the beginning. Since your body is used to getting its energy from glucose, it doesn't have enough of the enzymes used to convert fat into energy. Building up these enzymes takes a while, and that is why many people experience the keto flu or just generally feel tired when they start the keto diet.

The main aim of the ketogenic diet is to keep you in ketosis at all times. Depleting your body's glycogen stores and changing over to using ketones as the preferred energy source can take anything from four weeks to a couple of months. But, once you are fully keto-adapted, you will carry less water weight; your stamina and overall energy levels will increase; and you'll feel healthier in general. To allow your body to become fully keto-adapted, I recommend following a keto diet for at least sixty days.

If you're fat-fueled, you can up your daily carb allowance to up to 1.76 ounces a day without being kicked out of ketosis. Then again, if you do happen to eat too many carbs and your body switches over to glucose metabolism, it will be much easier to get back into ketosis the second time.

Keto Food Breakdown

Keto is low-carb, not no-carb. That is one thing to remember when building your perfect keto meal. There are three basic macronutrient splits to choose from—ranging from eating less than 20 grams of carbs to staying just under 100 grams—but these are guidelines and not hard-and-fast rules. I will cover the protein/fat/carbohydrate ratio later in this book. For now, let's look at what you may and may not eat.

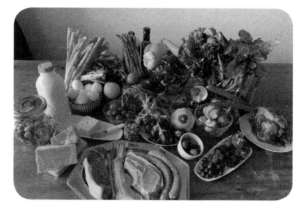

Good Foods to Eat

Meat

The ketogenic diet is not a high-protein diet, so you won't be required to buy a considerable amount of meat. The meat you buy should be unprocessed. Smoked and treated meat usually contain hidden sugar, which will stop your body from going into ketosis. If you want to check how much carbs are hidden in sausages, cold cuts, and other processed meats, just look at the label (if there is one). Anything below 5% carb content is okay, but if I were you, I'd avoid it altogether. Organic and grass-fed meat is healthiest, so opt for that whenever you have the choice.

Fish and Seafood

Fatty fish is the best. Salmon and tuna are great choices, or smaller fish like herring, mackerel, and sardines. Avoid fish that is covered in a crust as the carb content will be high.

Eggs

Eggs are a staple in the keto diet. One egg contains less than an ounce of carbohydrate but has a high protein content. Eggs are super versatile, and you can eat them any way you want on the keto diet. I am particularly fond of scrambled eggs with a healthy dose of butter and even some cream mixed in.

Vegetables

If your only introduction to keto has been photos on social media where the plate is packed with bacon, eggs, and cheese with no vegetables, then you've been misled.

Vegetables are essential as they contain a lot of vitamins and nutrients our bodies need to thrive. The only veggies you should avoid when following the keto diet are root vegetables as these contain more carbs. Beetroot, potatoes, carrots, and sweet potatoes are examples of vegetables to avoid.

Keto-friendly vegetables include lettuce, spinach, cabbage, cauliflower, kale, broccoli, avocado, and zucchini. You'll be interested to know that green vegetables usually contain fewer carbs than colorful veggies. Green bell peppers are a good example because they contain less carbs than red or yellow peppers.

You will notice that you'll end up eating more vegetables than when you weren't following the ketogenic diet. The reason is that vegetables replace the carbohydrates you'd usually fill your plate with, including pasta, rice, and potatoes. Actually, you'll soon see that cauliflower is so versatile, it can even transform into a pizza base!

Fruit

Fruit is notoriously high in sugar and carbs. In fact, you'll struggle to find any fruit other than berries that contain less than five percent carbohydrates. This unfortunately means that you'll be restricted to berries, and only within limits. What I like most about berries is their ability to get rid of any overwhelming sugar cravings—think of them as nature's candy.

Nuts

You're allowed to eat nuts on the keto diet, but you will have to keep in mind that they're fairly high-calorie. So, if you're explicitly following the keto diet to lose weight, eating too many nuts will make it easy to overshoot your calorie allowance for the day.

Avoid eating cashews as they're high in carbs; select macadamia, Brazil, or pecan nuts instead.

Full-Fat Dairy

Fat is your friend when you're following the keto diet, and all your dairy products should thus be full-fat. Milk, in general, should be used sparingly as the sugar in milk quickly adds to your daily carb allowance—there's 15 grams of carbs in one glass of milk! Choose cream over milk. When it comes to yogurt, full-fat and unsweetened is the way to go. If you buy low-fair flavored yogurt, you will be eating a lot of unnecessary sugar and less of the probiotic goodness you're hoping for.

Oil and High-Fat Condiments

When eating the keto way, you're getting most of your calories from fat. A lot of the fat will come from natural sources like meat, eggs, avocado, etc. But you'll also be using fat in your cooking—butter, coconut oil, and olive oil will regularly form part of recipes. Other than that, you can flavor your food with low-carb, high-fat sauces.

Bad Foods to Avoid

Sugary Foods

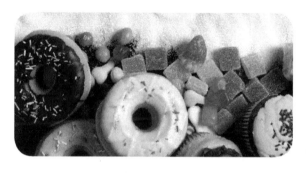

Sugar is a big no-no. Avoid any soft drinks, sports drinks, fruit juice, or flavored water. No cakes, cookies, chocolate, candy, or breakfast cereals are allowed. The best way to know is to read the label. If you see sugar, glucose, sucrose, or fructose on the label, avoid eating it.

I suggest you make it a habit of checking labels and looking at the sugar and carbohydrate content specifically. There are a lot of hidden sugars in food, especially drinks, sauces, condiments, and most packaged goods.

You can use artificial sweeteners, but limit how much you consume. They can have a negative influence on your health and may even slow down the weight-loss process. Instead, use some honey—sparingly.

Most, if not all, fruits fall in the "sugary food" category. Although I mentioned that berries are fine to eat in moderation, other fruits should be avoided. They're starchy, high in sugar, and not keto-friendly.

Starches

Breads, pasta, rice, oats, potatoes, muesli, whole grain products, and other starches should be avoided. This includes vegetables that grow underground. Similarly, beans and lentils are high in carbs; as a result, they're not allowed. There are some who argue that it is okay to treat yourself to non-refined starches such as legumes, potato, sweet potato, and other root vegetables from time to time, but that would depend on how much carbs your specific eating plan allows. For example, if you limit yourself to 15 percent of your macronutrients being carbs, it will be hard not to overshoot that if you eat carb-heavy food—even in moderation.

A Word of Caution

Since the ketogenic diet has gained popularity, a lot of food companies have jumped on the bandwagon in the hopes of cashing in on the craze. You'll find a lot of keto-friendly or low-carb products on the shelves, but the problem is these foods aren't always what the name suggests. Read the label and look for hidden carbohydrates, but more so, look for added additives like sugar alcohols and 'natural' sweeteners. A lot of the ingredients in such processed packaged foods are counterintuitive to weight loss since they may cause some metabolic issues. Keep that in mind. Natural is always best.

What's to Drink?

Don't worry, I'm not going to answer with 'water' and leave it there. Although water should be your number one option, sometimes we want something with a little more flavor. You can add sliced cucumbers, lemons, mint, or anything else that strikes your fancy to your water to make it taste like something, but if you're still looking for something else—coffee and tea are allowed! The only thing to remember is: no sugar. You can, however, add a bit of milk or cream.

If you feel you need an energy boost for the day ahead, make yourself what is known as bulletproof coffee. This mixture of coffee, butter, oil, and sometimes even cream will get you through the day. Some people will even forgo breakfast and drink a cup of bulletproof coffee instead. Just keep an eye on your weight; if your weight loss stalls, you may be drinking your calories and thus end up exceeding your calorie intake daily.

Bone broth is another drink that I recommend you keep handy. It's satisfying and contains a lot of nutrients, but more importantly, it will replace some of the electrolytes that you will inevitably lose on the keto diet.

The only drinks you have to avoid are ones that contain sugar, as mentioned earlier. And, of course, alcohol. The amount of sugar in some alcohol is staggering, and even if the alcohol contains no sugar, the fluid you mix it with certainly does. If you're out socializing and you feel the need to drink something, whiskey is the best choice—neat.

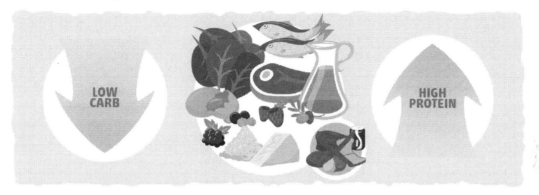

Macronutrients and Keto

If you follow the ketogenic diet, your macronutrients—that is, the fats, proteins, and carbohydrates—should be divided into 60% to 70% fat, 20% to 30% protein, and 5% to 10% carbs (Masood et al., 2020). That means you're looking at between 0.70 and 1.70 ounces of carbs a day.

The importance of getting the right balance of macronutrients can't be understated. It will make sure that your body gets all the essentials it needs to function. Each macronutrient contains a certain amount of energy (calories).

* Fat = 9 calories per 0.03 ounce
* Protein = 4 calories per 0.03 ounce
* Carbohydrate = 4 calories per 0.03 ounce

The exact amount of carbs to eat depends on your goals as well as your individual makeup. For instance, if you have type 2 diabetes, your blood glucose and insulin resistance will improve faster if you eat fewer carbohydrates. The same applies to when you're trying to lose weight. The only problem with eating so few carbs is that it is very restrictive, and you may find it challenging to stick to it. If that is the case, increasing your carbs may be the answer to your problem. Nevertheless, your daily carb intake should remain below 3.5 ounces for it to be considered a low-carb diet.

Keep in mind, the higher your daily carb consumption, the harder it will be for your body to go into ketosis. So, although you will be eating low-carb, you won't technically be following the ketogenic diet. Some staunch keto dieters will even argue that anything above 0.70 ounces of carbohydrates a day is not keto.

Let's look at a general breakdown of macronutrients for someone who is eating 2000 calories a day on a strict ketogenic diet.

*   70% fat = 5.48 ounces
*   20% protein = 4.40 ounces
*   10% carbohydrates = 1.73 ounces

It's also good to note that it's best to calculate only digestible carbs (net carbs). This means fiber is not added to your daily carb allowance, and you'll, in essence, be able to eat more carbohydrates. There are hundreds of macronutrient calculators on the internet or available for download for your phone. I recommend using one, especially in the beginning.

The Downsides of Ketosis

I mentioned the keto flu, which everyone starting the ketogenic diet dreads. Luckily, not everyone gets it. If you ate a lot of carbohydrates and were fairly inactive before starting the keto diet, the transition may be more of a shock to your body, and you're more likely to get the keto flu.

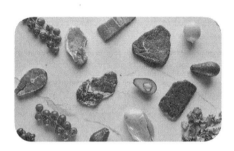

Symptoms can vary from mild to severe, and the duration of the flu depends on each person (Westman et al., 2008).

Indications that you have the keto flu are:

*   Nausea
*   Weakness
*   Constipation
*   Vomiting
*   Diarrhea
*   Stomach pain
*   Difficulty sleeping

*   Muscle cramps
*   Poor concentration
*   Headache
*   Muscle soreness
*   Irritability
*   Dizziness
*   Sugar cravings

There are ways to make keto flu more manageable, including drinking a lot of water and making sure you increase your electrolyte intake.

Another negative effect that the keto diet may have on you is increased stress levels. It's clear that switching between these two metabolic states is taxing on the body. At first, when your body realizes there is not enough glycogen to use as fuel, it will frantically start searching for an energy source. This will trigger the release of cortisol and other stress hormones. However, as soon as your body is keto-adapted, your body won't be under stress anymore and won't need to discharge cortisol.

At the beginning of your keto journey, you may also experience interrupted sleep. Although this is partly due to the increase of cortisol, lower levels of serotonin and melatonin are also to blame.

The science behind it comes down to not having a constant supply of L-tryptophan. Carbs help with the entry of this amino acid into the brain, and since that is in limited supply, your brain doesn't get enough L-tryptophan. This amino acid helps in the production of serotonin—a feel-good hormone, which in turn gets converted to melatonin—a sleep hormone.

You're able to buy L-tryptophan as a supplement to help you while your body is transitioning.

6 Keto Myths

Keto may come across as fairly straightforward: limit carbs, eat a lot of fat, and only eat some protein. But there are tons of misinformation that either over-simplify or, alternatively, complicate the ketogenic diet. Then, of course, you get the misinformation meant to scare people into not trying it.

1. It's all about eating a lot of fat

There is a misconception out there that fatty foods like bacon fried in butter are all you eat on a keto diet. If you go onto any social media platform and search for keto, you'll find thousands of photos brandishing plate after plate of food gleaming from the oil it was cooked in, and there's hardly ever a vegetable in sight. Unfortunately, this is the perfect fodder for people who are against the keto diet and claim it will clog your arteries.

To these people I say, vegetables are not optional when you're eating the keto way, and since you're only allowed to eat a certain percentage of fat a day, you can't drench your food and guzzle down butter and cream.

2. Keto will lead to ketoacidosis

Ketoacidosis is when both ketone levels and blood sugar are exceptionally high at the same time. This is more of a danger to people who have diabetes or have impaired liver function. However, if your pancreas is functioning normally, it's close to impossible to achieve ketoacidosis.

Normal ketosis has a ketone level of 3 mmol/L and low blood sugar, while ketoacidosis registers 30 mmol/L or more ketones and high blood sugar levels.

If you're unsure if you're in danger of developing ketoacidosis, talk to your doctor before starting the keto diet.

3. All fat is bad fat

There's this idea that fat will make you fat and eventually lead to your death. If you eat only trans fats, I would wholeheartedly agree. Man-made fats are bad for your health; however, the keto diet calls for eating healthy, high-quality natural fats. If you eat fats that are good for you, you will feel satiated for longer, meaning the likelihood of you binging on carbs is reduced.

If it's your cholesterol, you're worried about, don't be. Good fats actually lower harmful cholesterol while contributing to your heart health. If you eat too little fat, your cholesterol may be extra low, and that is not healthy either. Research done over the years found that the ketogenic diet is actually healthier and more effective in weight loss and improving overall health than a low-fat diet (Manikam, 2008).

Apart from being good for your heart and brain, good-quality fat lowers inflammation, helps for depression and anxiety, and regulates fat-burning hormones.

4. Keto will cause liver damage

Some people are concerned that the fat intake that is part of the keto diet will cause fatty deposits in the liver, which will lead to fatty liver disease or nonalcoholic steatohepatitis. However, for this to happen, four things must occur in the body at the same time.

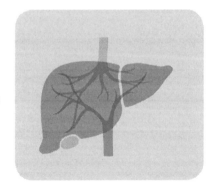

* Insulin resistance
* Extreme fat-burning
* High inflammation
* Oxidative stress

At the beginning of the ketogenic diet, numbers one, three, and four start improving as soon as sugar consumption stops, and the person starts eating and living healthily. Of course, it's not going to happen overnight.

Since the fat-burning process is only in full force later on, the person will be much healthier in general, and only number two will be in play.

5. Keto is bad for your kidneys

This is a widespread myth. The two main drivers of this myth are the belief that a person will develop kidney stones due to the high protein intake and that an increased acidity of the urine will cause kidney stress.

After what you read so far, it should be obvious that kidney stones should not be a concern since keto is not a high-protein diet.

When it comes to increased urine acidity, that is only a problem if you suffer from ketoacidosis and not nutritional ketosis.

In actual fact, a diet high in carbohydrates is much more likely to damage a person's kidneys (Nam, 2019).

6. Keto increases your risk of heart disease

It's true, keto can raise your cholesterol. But, it's not that simple.

Firstly, cholesterol has a bad rap for causing heart disease, but all the good it does is often overlooked. It is necessary for a lot of critical bodily functions, including the production of bile and the creation of estrogen, progesterone, testosterone, and other hormones, among other duties. So, lowering your cholesterol may not be all that good for your body to perform vital processes.

Cholesterol is often just thought of as one thing, when there are actually good (HDL) and bad (LDL) cholesterol, and even the LDL has two types—patterns A and B. Pattern B is small and dense, and it's the dangerous type that clings to the walls of our arteries and causes damage.

What most people don't know is that plant-based processed oils (as opposed to animal oils and fats used on the keto diet) may reduce your LDL cholesterol, but it is, in reality, LDL A which gets broken down, while the dangerous pattern B increases—and with it so does your risk of heart disease.

As you can see, not all fats are equal.

Tips to Guarantee Your Success

Follow these tips, and you'll be well on your way to turning your body into a fat-burning machine.

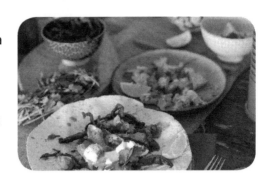

1. Low-carb is key
Your carb intake should not exceed 1.70 ounces a day. The fewer carbs you eat, the faster you will enter ketosis and become fat-adapted.

2. Get active
Physical activity is not only good for weight loss; it is good for your heart too. If you exercise while transitioning from glucose metabolism to ketosis, you will deplete your body's glycogen stores faster than you would without physical activity. This means your body will be forced to start burning fat for fuel sooner.

3. Eat enough protein
Don't neglect your protein intake. Protein not only preserves muscle, but also helps to build muscle. I'm not saying you should overdo it, but keep it to 30% to 35% of your daily macronutrient intake.

4. Clean out your pantry
This is very important. If you only have keto-friendly food in your home, you won't be able to cheat when a carb craving strikes. Stocking your pantry with keto snacks is not a good idea if you struggle to control yourself.

5. Plan your meals ahead of time
If you have a plan to stick to, it will be more difficult to deviate from it. You can meal-prep for a whole week, or you can use your Instant Pot to cook a keto-friendly meal. You'll be less tempted to make a quick stop at your favorite take-out if you know there's a healthy and warm meal containing just the right macronutrients waiting for you at home.

I think it's time for me to introduce you to the Instant Pot (if you don't already own one).

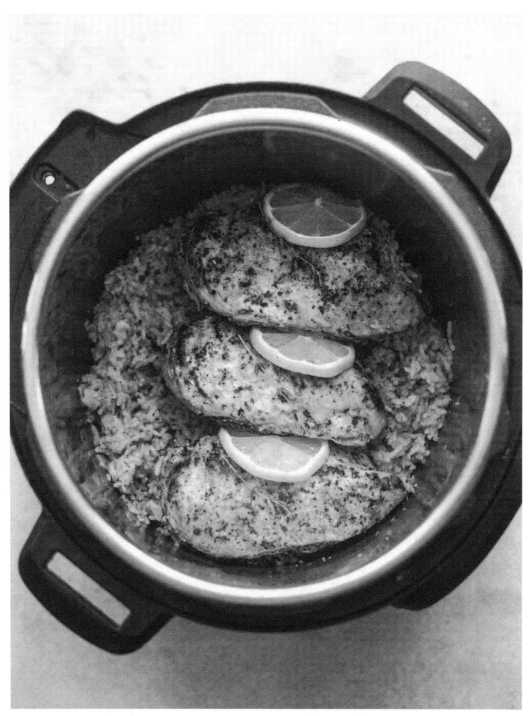

CHAPTER 2
Instant Pot 101

What makes the Instant Pot such a great kitchen appliance is its versatility—it's not just an electric pressure cooker, but also a slow cooker, a rice maker, a steamer, and in some models, a yogurt maker!

Since the steam inside the Instant Pot cannot escape, it creates a pressurized environment with a higher cooking temperature. You'll be able to cook delicious meals in half the time it would take on a traditional stovetop.

I am particularly fond of the timer function. Before I go to work in the morning, I add the keto-friendly ingredients to the pot and set the timer to start cooking an hour or two before I'll get home. That means I will come back to the mouth-watering aroma of whatever keto meal I decided on that morning.

But that's not the only reason why an Instant Pot and keto make the perfect pair.

Advantages of Using the Instant Pot for Keto Meals

For me, the appeal of cooking healthy meals in a fraction of the time was a big selling point when I first got my Instant Pot. This didn't change after I started the keto diet. But there are more reasons why this appliance is one of the most-used in my kitchen.

Safety first

The Instant Pot's built-in safety features make it more secure than a traditional pressure cooker. For example, if the lid is not tightly secured, the pot will not work.

Easy to clean

Not only do you have minimal dishes to do when you use an Instant Pot, the dishes you have to wash are easy to clean. In fact, most of the parts are dishwasher safe.

One of my favorite dishes to make is my grandma's one-pot chicken stew I adapted to keto—I just replaced the starchy vegetables like carrot and potato with zucchini and cauliflower and added some crispy bacon bits. If I were to make this on a stovetop, I'd have two pots, and a pan to clean!

Nutrients aren't lost

The longer you cook food, the more of the vitamins and minerals seep out into the air and water, which makes the Instant Pot a good choice to lock in all the goodness. Since the cooking time is so much shorter, you won't lose any of the nutritious value of the food.

This also means your food will have more flavor. On the stovetop, food gets superheated, which affects the taste profile. You will soon come to realize that the flavors of food cooked under pressure are so much more appetizing.

Kills germs

You never know what invisible nasties you're bringing home with you from the grocery store, especially on meat. You can rinse it when you get home, but some of these bacteria cling to the meat for dear life. But, when you use an Instant Pot, the food is cooked under high pressure at a lower temperature—conditions not conducive to bacteria and germ survival.

This is especially important considering that you will be eating a lot of chicken on the keto diet, and chicken is notorious for being contaminated with salmonella and E.coli. Even spinach has a bad rap for containing bacteria. Luckily now you won't have to worry about it!

It's effortless

Cooking with an Instant Pot is totally hands-off. You don't have to keep watch that nothing burns or boils over. There's no unnecessary stirring. All you do is put the ingredients in the pot, select the correct setting, and let the pot work its magic.

Some other reasons why the Instant Pot is an instant hit in my books:

✳ You don't need to sauté food.
✳ It's heat efficient.
✳ Suitable for use when traveling or in small spaces such as RVs, dorm rooms, etc.

That brings me to my next point: choosing a cooker that fits your needs.

What Size Instant Pot Should I Get?

The answer to this comes down to one thing—how many people are you cooking for. There are various makes and models available on the market, but they all come in three sizes: 3 quart, 6 quart, and 8 quarts.

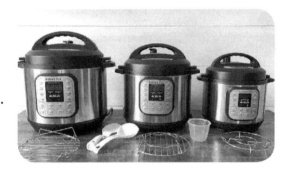

The standard size of most Instant Pots you'll find in the store are 6 quarts, and you'll be able to comfortably feed up to six people with this size. But, if you only want to cook for two, then getting a 3-quart pot is best.

For large families or if you fancy yourself an entertainer, get the 8-quart size.

I also suggest you think about what you plan on cooking. Since you're following the ketogenic diet, you won't need presets like making rice, cooking porridge, and baking cake (unless it's a keto-friendly cake). So, look at the functions on the specific Instant Pot you have your eye on and consider if you're actually going to use them, or if you're just wasting your money and a cheaper cooker will do the job.

The Buttons

Let's look at what the general buttons on an Instant Pot do. Keep in mind that the buttons you see depend on the model of Instant Pot you have.

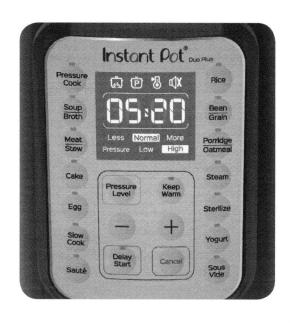

Sauté

Used to brown onions or meat. Press the Sauté button and wait for a beep that indicates your cooker has reached the temperature you selected. If you want to toggle between temperatures, press the Adjust button if there is one; if not, press the Sauté button again.

Manual or pressure cook

Depending on the type of pot you have, you will see either a Manual or Pressure Cook button on the machine's control panel. This is what you press if you want to pressure cook. The pressure is usually automatically set to high, but if that is not the case, there should be pressure level buttons you can use to adjust the pressure.

Setting the cooking time

Press plus or minus to set the desired cooking time. Wait a few seconds, and 'On' will display on the screen. This means your Instant Pot is now ready to pressurize. After the cooking process is complete and the time has run out, L0:00 or 0:00 will appear on the screen. The 'L' stands for lapsed time. The timer will now start to count up to show the time lapsed between the cooking ending and complete pressure release.

Keep warm/cancel

This is pretty self-explanatory—a setting to keep your food warm. Some models have the Keep Warm/Cancel buttons as one. The Cancel button is used to switch between functions or to switch the cooker off when done using it. After pressing it, wait for 'Off' to appear on the screen to make sure your Instant Pot is safely switched off.

Delay Start

One of my favorite functions. Pressing this button will delay the cooking process. You can prep all the food in the pot and set the timer to start a few hours before you want to eat. This is especially great if you want to come home to a cooked meal after a day at the office. Just keep in mind that meat cannot be left out of the fridge for too long.

The Icons

If you bought a pot with a digital display, you'll see various icons light up and specific times.

* **Flame under a pot:** The pot is busy heating.
* **'P' in a pot:** The pot is set to "Pressure Cook".
* **Thermometer:** The pot keeping food warm.
* **Speaker with an 'X' next to it:** Sound is muted. In fact, there may come a time when the sound becomes annoying, and you want to turn it off. If you own a Duo, Duo Plus, Duo Nova, SV, or Viva model, all you have to do is press the minus button until the machine displays 'SOff'. To turn the sound on again, press the plus button until you see 'SOn'.

On the Ultra and Duo Evo Plus models, while 'Off' is on the screen, press and hold the knob for a few seconds. Turn the knob to select the setting you prefer and press the knob again for a few seconds to lock the setting in place.

Lid and Trivet

A super space-saving functionality is the option to put the lid in an upright position. There are two slides on the lid that slot into to open rectangles on the pot. This means you can place the lid upright while sautéing to save counter space!

If you place the lid in this position, keep in mind that you have to lift the lid up and place it on the pot to close it. There is no hinge mechanism. I don't want you to break the plastic on the sides of the lid because you thought you could just flip the lid closed.

The trivet is a wire rack that comes with most Instant Pots. It's a useful way to cook two dishes at the same time. Let's say you're cooking meat in a sauce at the bottom of the pot. Instead of waiting for the meat to be done before you start cooking the vegetables, you can place the veggies in a separate dish on the trivet over the meat.

Pressure/Steam Release

The pressure/steam release has a dual purpose. Firstly, when the Instant Pot's pressure release setting is set to 'sealing,' the pot will be able to start building pressure. For this to happen, the lid needs to be securely in place.

As soon as the cooking time is over, you can change the pressure release to 'venting,' which will allow steam to escape in preparation for you to open the pot.

There are three different ways to depressurize the cooker. You will need to know the difference between each as the method will not be the same for all recipes.

A **quick pressure release (QPR)** is where you allow all the steam to escape at once. This method is great to use when you're preparing veggies or other foods that don't require a lot of time to cook.

If you leave the cooker to lose its pressure naturally as it cools down, you're using the **natural pressure release (NPR)** method. This process can take anything from a few minutes to 30 minutes or even longer—it depends on the pressure selection and the volume of food in the pot.

Timed natural release is when you let pressure escape naturally for 10 to 15 minutes before venting the remaining steam at once. Using a timed NPR means steam won't release in such a geyser-like fashion as with just NPR.

Things to Remember Before Using Your Instant Pot

Although the Instant Pot is simple to use, it's not as easy as just plugging it into the power socket. There are a few things you will have to do to get your pot to work.

Liquid is Essential

Steam is the driving force behind an Instant Pot—and without water or another liquid, there won't be any. The fluid in the cooker releases vapor, but since it can't escape, pressure rises. That, combined with the constant low heat, is what cooks the food. A cup is usually all you need to get the process started. You will, however, find recipes that contain less liquid, but these dishes usually won't require pressurization to cook.

Don't Forget to Deglaze

When you sauté vegetables or meat, there will inevitably be some bits of food that will stick to the pot. To make sure that these food particles don't end up burning, add some water, and scrape the bottom of the pot with a wooden or silicone spoon. This is called deglazing, and a lot of recipes will require you to do this after any sautéing.

Always Cook In the Inner Pot

You may think this goes without saying, but you may get so caught up in a recipe that you end up adding ingredients before putting in place the stainless-steel inner pot. This will damage your Instant Pot and will be a waste of ingredients since everything will just trickle out of the bottom of the Instant Pot.

Don't Place Your Cooker On the Stove

I know some of us have small kitchens with limited counter space but resist the urge to place your Instant Pot on the stove. Accidents happen, and you may have the misfortune of turning on the burner by mistake and ruining your cooker.

Safety and Care Tips

To ensure that your Instant Pot is with you for a long time and stays in good working order, correct cleaning is probably the best thing you can do to prolong its use.

- After every use, rinse the sealing ring. Since it is dishwasher safe, you can add it for a deep clean. The sealing rings often absorb strong smells, so if you've been cooking curry, seafood, or any other pungent food, you may want to soak the sealing ring in some vinegar and steam it afterward.
- Remove the liner pot and use warm soapy water to wipe off any visible stains. If there are stains or food bits stuck in hard-to-reach areas, a Q-tip or toothbrush will help you clean those spots.
- The lid has a steam release valve and an anti-block shield that can easily be removed. Soak all elements and the lid itself in some warm foamy water. You can also wash these in a dishwasher.
- Once you've cleaned all the various components, let the all parts dry and reassemble your Instant Pot.

When it comes to safety, there are a few things you have to keep in mind.

- Double-check that the inner pot and heating plate are clean and dry.
- Make sure the float valve, exhaust valve, and anti-block shield have no food stuck to them.
- Secure the sealing ring.
- Check that the steam release valve is in the 'Sealing' position.
- Do not overfill the cooker. Foods that foam should not pass the halfway mark and other dishes should not fill the pot more than three-quarters.
- Use caution when releasing steam.
- Unplug your Instant Pot when not in use.
- Don't run any electrical parts of the appliance under water as you would when cooking with a traditional pressure cooker.
- If you double a recipe, don't double the cooking time.

Accessorize Your Instant Pot

You don't absolutely have to have these accessories for your Instant Pot, but it will make your cooking experience much more enjoyable.

Extra inner pot: If you store leftovers straight in the inner pot, get another one so that you won't get frustrated if you want to cook, but there's no clean inner pot.

Extra silicone rings: The more you use your Instant Pot, the quicker you will need to replace the silicone ring. Also, as mentioned earlier, it may be a good idea to keep specific silicone rings for foods with strong odors. They come in different colors, so you can color code based on sweet, savory, and seafood dishes.

Glass lid: Great to use when you're slow-cooking or heating food.

Silicone lid: A silicone lid secures tightly over the inner pot, meaning you don't have to decant into another container but can store as is.

Gripper clips: Don't get burned! Invest in gripper clips to ensure your safety.

Foil sling: A foil sling will make it possible to easily lift a casserole or cake pan out of the cooker. If you plan on doing a lot of pot-in-pot cooking, this is a must.

4-Ounce ramekins: Perfect for baked eggs, mini meatloaf, or delicious keto-friendly desserts such as deconstructed tiramisu.

1-Quart casserole dish: Cheesy, steamed veggies, or what about cauliflower lasagna? I highly recommend owning a casserole dish; you will use it a lot.

Steamer basket: Great if you loved steamed fish.

Steamer pans: I use steamer pans to reheat more than one dish in my cooker.

Springform pan: Mmmm, can you say cheesecake? A 7-inch pan will fit in a 6-quart or 8-quart Instant Pot.

Egg steamer rack: You'll be eating a lot of eggs on keto. To prevent eggs rolling around and cracking while hard-boiling, get yourself an egg steamer rack.

Frequently Asked Questions

I know it can be somewhat scary when you first use an Instant Pot. We've all heard scary stories of traditional pressure cookers exploding, and although we know the Instant Pot has added safety features, a lot of us are still overly cautious.

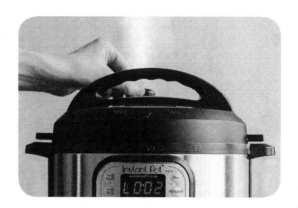

I hope these answers will prevent any frights when you first start using your Instant Pot.

1.Is the Instant Pot safe?

This cooker is nothing like the traditional stovetop pressure cookers our grandmas used. It has built-in safety features that include shut-off fuses, automatic pressure controls, lid locks, temperature controls, and protection from overheating.

If something is wrong, the pot will shut off and flash an error code.

2.My pot is plugged in but not working.

This happened to me before, and all I had to do was double-check that the cord was in place at the socket, as well as at the back of the Instant Pot.

3.What is PIP?

If you ever want to make keto cheesecake, this is the method you'll use! Pot-in-pot cooking is when you place a separate dish inside the pot, resting on top of a steam rack. The extra pot won't be submerged in the water but will instead be just above water level.

4.Can I cook food while still frozen?

Food like vegetables and smaller cuts of meat can be cooked from frozen, but you should remember to add extra cooking time to include the thawing process. The only real downside of cooking food that has not been defrosted is that it will not cook evenly, especially if we're talking about large pieces of meat. So, although it is technically possible to cook from frozen, I recommend thawing food beforehand.

5.After selecting a cooking program, nothing happens.

I know we're so eager to get cooking that we want everything to start immediately! However, in this case, there will be a 10-second delay after you select a specific function. This is to give you time to adjust any settings or to change the pressure.

6.Why is steam escaping from the sides while pressure cooking?

The silicone ring is not placed securely in the groove under the lid.

7.Why is the pot spraying water everywhere during quick release?

Don't panic; nothing is going to blow up! This happens when you overfill the pot with liquid, or if you cook a lot of starchy foods—which won't be happening since you're eating keto, right?

8.How long does it take for the pot to come to pressure?

If a recipe says a dish will take 10 minutes to cook, it doesn't mean the whole process will be done in that time. Think of your Instant Pot as an oven that needs to preheat. Similarly, it can take anything from 10 to 30 minutes for your pot to pressurize. It depends on how much liquid and food are in the pot. One trick is to use warm liquid; it will speed up the process considerably.

9.Why is the Instant Pot making clicking noises while cooking?

There are two reasons this may be happening. Firstly, the inner pot is wet on the outside. Check that the inner pot is completely dry on the outside before you put it in the cooker. Secondly, the cooker is regulating its temperature through power switching. This is nothing to worry about!

10.Do I need to double the cooking time when I double a recipe?

The cooking time isn't dependent on weight but rather the density of food, so you don't need to increase the cooking time. The only thing I suggest you keep in mind is that the pot will take longer to come to pressure if there are more ingredients in it.

11.What is a water test?

If you're new to cooking with an Instant Pot, this is a great way to get a feel of which buttons to press and how to do a pressure release. It's basically just a way to test if everything is in working order and to help put you at ease before you start cooking. But it isn't a necessary step to do beforehand.

Keto Food Cooking Sheet

I don't think people realize how fast cooking with an Instant Pot truly is until they see the cooking times. Below is how long it will take you to prepare foods you'll be enjoying a lot of on the keto diet.

Food	Cooking Times
Meat, Fish & Eggs	
Beef stew	20 min (per 1lb)
Beef large	20-25 min (per 1lb)
Beef ribs	20-25 min (per 1lb)
Chicken whole	8 min (per 1lb)
Chicken breasts	6-8 min (per 1lb)
Chicken bone stock	40-45 min (per 1lb)
Lamb leg	15 min (per 1lb)
Pork roast	15 min (per 1lb)
Pork baby back ribs	15-20 min (per 1lb)
Fish whole	4-5 min
Fish fillet	2-3 min
Lobster	2-3 min
Shrimp	1-3 min
Seafood stock	7-8 min
Eggs	5 min

Vegetables

Asparagus	1-2 min
Broccoli	1-2 min
Brussel sprouts	2-3 min
Cabbage (whole)	2-3 min
Cauliflower (florets)	2-3 min
Mixed vegetables	3-4 min

Now that you know how to use your Instant Pot to cook delectable keto meals, I think it is time that I share some of my much-loved recipes with you. Most, if not all, of these recipes are such favorites, my friends and family who aren't even on the keto diet always beg me to share some with them.

Don't forget, you can adapt any recipe and make it keto! Just remove all the starchy foods and replace it with keto-friendly vegetables. Go ahead and experiment. Who knows, maybe you're the next top chef of the keto Instant Pot world.

I hope all recipes in this book are a hit with your loved ones too. You will, above all, shock them if you prepare a healthy keto-friendly dessert—they won't believe that you're allowed to eat such yummy sweet dishes while you're on a 'diet.'

Who knows, maybe you can use our Instant Pot cooking to convince people to eat keto and live a healthier and prolonged life!

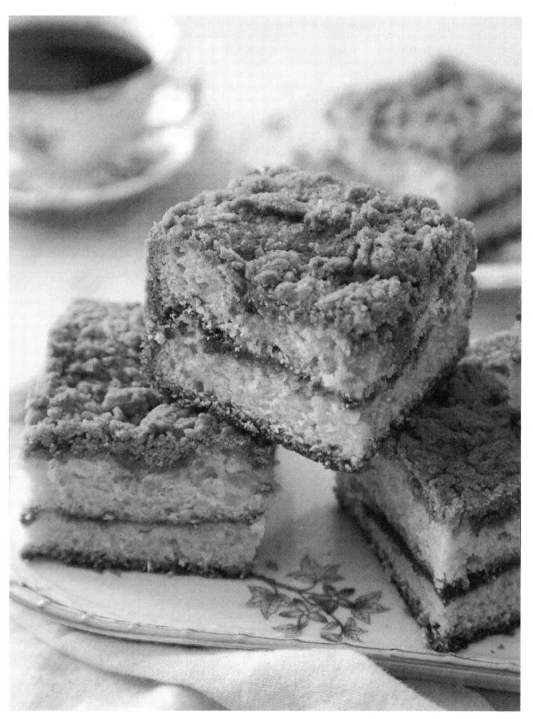

CHAPTER 3

Breakfasts

Bacon and Mushroom Quiche Lorraine

Prep time: 10 minutes | Cook time: 37 minutes | Serves 4

- 4 strips bacon, chopped
- 2 cups sliced button mushrooms
- ½ cup diced onions
- 8 large eggs
- 1½ cups shredded Swiss cheese
- 1 cup unsweetened almond milk
- ¼ cup sliced green onions
- ½ teaspoon sea salt
- ¼ teaspoon ground black pepper
- 2 tablespoons coconut flour

1. Press the Sauté button on the Instant Pot and add the bacon. Sauté for 4 minutes, or until crisp. Transfer the bacon to a plate lined with paper towel to drain, leaving the drippings in the pot.
2. Add the mushrooms and diced onions to the pot and sauté for 3 minutes, or until the onions are tender. Remove the mixture from the pot to a large bowl. Wipe the Instant Pot clean.
3. Set a trivet in the Instant Pot and pour in 1 cup water.
4. In a medium bowl, stir together the eggs, cheese, almond milk, green onions, salt and pepper. Pour the egg mixture into the bowl with the mushrooms and onions. Stir to combine. Fold in the coconut flour. Pour the mixture into a greased round casserole dish. Spread the cooked bacon on top.
5. Place the casserole dish onto the trivet in the Instant Pot.
6. Lock the lid, select the Manual mode and set the cooking time for 30 minutes on High Pressure. When the timer goes off, do a natural pressure release for 15 minutes, then release any remaining pressure. Open the lid.
7. Remove the casserole dish from the Instant Pot.
8. Let cool for 15 to 30 minutes before cutting into 4 pieces. Serve immediately.

Per Serving

calories: 433 | fat: 29.1g | protein: 32.0g | carbs: 6.9g | net carbs: 4.8g | fiber: 2.1g

Easy Eggs Benedict

Prep time: 5 minutes | Cook time: 1 minute | Serves 3

- 1 teaspoon butter
- 3 eggs
- ¼ teaspoon salt
- ½ teaspoon ground black pepper
- 1 cup water
- 3 turkey bacon slices, fried

1. Grease the eggs molds with the butter and crack the eggs inside. Sprinkle with salt and ground black pepper.
2. Pour the water and insert the trivet in the Instant Pot. Put the eggs molds on the trivet.
3. Set the lid in place. Select the Manual mode and set the cooking time for 1 minute on High Pressure. When the timer goes off, do a quick pressure release. Carefully open the lid.
4. Transfer the eggs onto the plate. Top the eggs with the fried bacon slices.

Per Serving

calories: 94 | fat: 6.1g | protein: 8.7g | carbs: 0.5g | net carbs: 0.4g | fiber: 0.1g

Broccoli, Ham, and Pepper Frittata

Prep time: 10 minutes | Cook time: 20 minutes | Serves 4

- ❀ 1 cup sliced bell peppers
- ❀ 8 ounces (227 g) ham, cubed
- ❀ 2 cups frozen broccoli florets
- ❀ 4 eggs
- ❀ 1 cup heavy cream
- ❀ 1 cup grated Cheddar cheese
- ❀ 1 teaspoon salt
- ❀ 2 teaspoons freshly ground black pepper

1. Arrange the pepper slices in a greased pan. Place the cubed ham on top. Cover with the frozen broccoli.
2. In a bowl, whisk together the remaining ingredients. Pour the egg mixture over the vegetables and ham. Cover the pan with aluminum foil.
3. Pour 2 cups water and insert the trivet in the Instant Pot. Put the pan on the trivet.
4. Lock the lid. Select the Manual mode and set the cooking time for 20 minutes on High Pressure. Once the timer goes off, perform a natural pressure release for 10 minutes, then release any remaining pressure. Carefully open the lid.
5. Carefully remove the pan from the pot and remove the foil. Let the frittata sit for 5 to 10 minutes before transferring the frittata onto the plate.
6. Serve warm.

Per Serving
calories: 395 | fat: 26.8g | protein: 30.1g | carbs: 8.8g | net carbs: 5.7g | fiber: 3.1g

Gruyère Asparagus Frittata

Prep time: 10 minutes | Cook time: 22 minutes | Serves 6

- ❀ 6 eggs
- ❀ 6 tablespoons heavy cream
- ❀ ½ teaspoon salt
- ❀ ½ teaspoon black pepper
- ❀ 1 tablespoon butter
- ❀ 2½ ounces (71 g) asparagus, chopped
- ❀ 1 clove garlic, minced
- ❀ 1¼ cup shredded Gruyère cheese, divided
- ❀ Cooking spray
- ❀ 3 ounces (85 g) halved cherry tomatoes
- ❀ ½ cup water

1. In a large bowl, stir together the eggs, cream, salt, and pepper.
2. Set the Instant Pot on the Sauté mode and melt the butter. Add the asparagus and garlic to the pot and sauté for 2 minutes, or until the garlic is fragrant. The asparagus should still be crisp.
3. Transfer the asparagus and garlic to the bowl with the egg mixture. Stir in 1 cup of the cheese. Clean the pot.
4. Spritz a baking pan with cooking spray. Spread the tomatoes in a single layer in the pan. Pour the egg mixture on top of the tomatoes and sprinkle with the remaining ¼ cup of the cheese. Cover the pan tightly with aluminum foil.
5. Pour the water in the Instant Pot and insert the trivet. Place the pan on the trivet.
6. Set the lid in place. Select the Manual mode and set the cooking time for 20 minutes on High Pressure. When the timer goes off, perform a quick pressure release. Carefully open the lid.
7. Remove the pan from the pot and remove the foil. Blot off any excess moisture with a paper towel. Let the frittata cool for 5 to 10 minutes before transferring onto a plate.

Per Serving
calories: 204 | fat: 16.6g | protein: 11.3g | carbs: 2.2g | net carbs: 1.6g | fiber: 0.6g

Flavor-Packed Breakfast Pizza

Prep time: 15 minutes | Cook time: 20 minutes | Serves 4 to 5

- 2 tablespoons avocado oil
- 1 pound (454 g) ground chicken
- ¼ cup water
- ½ teaspoon crushed red pepper
- ½ teaspoon freshly ground black pepper
- ½ teaspoon dried parsley
- ½ teaspoon kosher salt
- ½ teaspoon dried basil
- 1 (14-ounce / 397-g) can unsweetened crushed tomatoes, drained
- 1 cup shredded Cheddar cheese
- 2 to 4 slices bacon, cooked and finely cut

1. Press the Sauté button on the Instant Pot and melt the avocado oil. Add the ground chicken to the pot and sauté for 5 minutes, or until browned. Pour in the water. Push the chicken down with a spatula to form a flat, even layer, covering the bottom of the pot.
2. In a small bowl, stir together the red pepper, black pepper, parsley, salt and basil.
3. Spread the tomatoes over the chicken. Add a layer of cheese and then the bacon. Top with the spice and herb mixture.
4. Lock the lid. Select the Manual mode and set the cooking time for 15 minutes on High Pressure. Once the timer goes off, perform a natural pressure release for 10 minutes, then release any remaining pressure. Carefully open the lid.
5. Remove the pizza with a spatula. Serve hot.

Per Serving

calories: 173 | fat: 11.6g | protein: 10.2g | carbs: 8.7g | net carbs: 6.3g | fiber: 2.4g

Kale and Sausage Egg Muffins

Prep time: 5 minutes | Cook time: 9 to 10 minutes | Serves 2

- 3 teaspoons avocado oil, divided
- 4 ounces (113 g) fully cooked chicken sausage, diced
- 4 small kale leaves, finely chopped
- ½ teaspoon kosher salt, divided
- ½ teaspoon ground black pepper, divided
- 4 large eggs
- ¼ cup heavy whipping cream
- 1 cup water

1. Grease the bottom and insides of four silicone muffin cups with 1 teaspoon of the avocado oil.
2. Press the Sauté button on the Instant Pot and heat the remaining 2 teaspoons of the avocado oil. Add the sausage to the pot and sauté for 2 minutes. Add the chopped kale and ¼ teaspoon of the salt and black pepper. Sauté for 2 to 3 minutes, or until the kale is wilted.
3. Meanwhile, in a medium bowl, lightly whisk together the eggs, cream and the remaining ¼ teaspoon of the salt and pepper.
4. Divide the kale and sausage mixture among the four muffin cups. Pour the egg mixture evenly over the kale and sausage and stir lightly with a fork. Loosely cover the cups with foil.
5. Pour the water and insert the trivet in the Instant Pot. Put the muffin cups on the trivet.
6. Lock the lid. Select the Manual mode and set the cooking time for 5 minutes on High Pressure. Once the timer goes off, perform a natural pressure release for 10 minutes, then release any remaining pressure. Carefully open the lid.
7. Remove the muffins from the Instant Pot. Serve hot.

Per Serving

calories: 389 | fat: 32.9g | protein: 19.1g | carbs: 3.4g | net carbs: 3.1g | fiber: 0.3g

Chorizo and Egg Lettuce Tacos

Prep time: 5 minutes | Cook time: 12 minutes | Serves 6

- ✿ 2 tablespoons avocado oil
- ✿ 1½ pounds (680 g) fresh chorizo
- ✿ ¾ cup sour cream
- ✿ ½ cup chicken broth
- ✿ 6 large eggs, washed
- ✿ 6 large lettuce leaves

1. Press the Sauté button on the Instant Pot and heat the oil. Crumble in the chorizo. Sauté for 2 minutes, breaking up the meat with a wooden spoon or meat chopper.
2. Stir in the sour cream and broth.
3. Place a long-legged metal trivet directly on top of the sausage mixture. Place the eggs on the trivet.
4. Set the lid in place. Select the Manual mode and set the cooking time for 10 minutes on High Pressure.
5. Meanwhile, fill a medium bowl with ice water for the eggs.
6. When the timer goes off, do a quick pressure release. Carefully open the lid.
7. Use tongs or a large spoon to transfer the eggs immediately to the ice bath. Stir the chorizo mixture and allow it to rest in the Instant Pot on Keep Warm.
8. When the eggs are cool enough to handle, peel and slice them.
9. To serve, use a slotted spoon to spoon the chorizo into lettuce leaves.

Per Serving

calories: 671 | fat: 55.9g | protein: 35.0g | carbs: 4.9g | net carbs: 4.7g | fiber: 0.2g

Almond Butter Beef Bowl

Prep time: 10 minutes | Cook time: 7 minutes | Serves 4

- ✿ 1 tablespoon avocado oil
- ✿ 1 pound (454 g) ground beef
- ✿ 1 clove garlic, minced
- ✿ ½ teaspoon sea salt
- ✿ ½ teaspoon ground black pepper
- ✿ ½ teaspoon ground turmeric
- ✿ ¼ teaspoon ground cinnamon
- ✿ ¼ teaspoon ground coriander
- ✿ ¼ cup almond butter
- ✿ ½ cup full-fat coconut milk
- ✿ 1 small head green cabbage, shredded

1. Press the Sauté button on the Instant Pot and heat the oil. Crumble in the ground beef and cook for 3 minutes, breaking up the meat with a wooden spoon or meat chopper.
2. Stir in the garlic, salt, black pepper, turmeric, cinnamon, and coriander.
3. Add the almond butter and coconut milk. Stir constantly until the almond butter melts and mixes with the coconut milk. Layer the cabbage on top of the meat mixture but do not stir.
4. Set the lid in place. Select the Manual mode and set the cooking time for 4 minutes on High Pressure. When the timer goes off, do a quick pressure release. Carefully open the lid.
5. Stir the meat mixture. Taste and adjust the salt and black pepper, and add more red pepper flakes if desired. Use a slotted spoon to transfer the mixture to a serving bowl. Serve hot.

Per Serving

calories: 534 | fat: 43.2g | protein: 26.4g | carbs: 15.0g | net carbs: 9.2g | fiber: 5.8g

Pumpkin Cake with Walnuts

Prep time: 5 minutes | Cook time: 40 minutes | Serves 5 to 6

✿ 1 cup water

Base:

✿ 3 eggs
✿ 1 cup almond flour
✿ ¾ cup chopped walnuts
✿ ½ cup organic pumpkin purée
✿ ¼ cup heavy whipping cream
✿ 2 tablespoons butter, softened
✿ ½ teaspoon ground cinnamon
✿ ½ teaspoon ground nutmeg
✿ ½ teaspoon baking powder
✿ ½ teaspoon salt

Topping:

✿ ¼ cup heavy whipping cream
✿ ½ cup Swerve
✿ ½ cup unsweetened coconut flakes

1. Pour the water and insert the trivet in the Instant Pot.
2. Using an electric mixer, combine all the ingredients for the cake. Mix thoroughly. Transfer the mixture into a well-greased baking pan.
3. Place the pan onto the trivet and cover loosely with aluminum foil.
4. Lock the lid. Select the Manual mode and set the cooking time for 40 minutes on High Pressure.
5. Meanwhile, in a large bowl, whisk together all the ingredients for the topping.
6. Once the timer goes off, perform a natural pressure release for 10 minutes, then release any remaining pressure. Carefully open the lid.
7. Remove the pan from the pot. Sprinkle the topping mixture evenly over the cake. Let cool for 5 minutes before serving.

Per Serving

calories: 333 | fat: 30.5g | protein: 7.9g | carbs: 7.8g | net carbs: 3.0g | fiber: 4.8g

Peppery Ham Frittata

Prep time: 10 minutes | Cook time: 40 minutes | Serves 2

- ✿ 2 tablespoons avocado oil, divided
- ✿ ¼ cup chopped onion
- ✿ ¼ cup chopped green bell pepper
- ✿ ¼ cup chopped red bell pepper
- ✿ ½ pound (227 g) cooked ham, cubed
- ✿ 6 large eggs
- ✿ ½ cup heavy whipping cream
- ✿ ½ teaspoon sea salt
- ✿ ¼ teaspoon ground black pepper
- ✿ ¼ teaspoon dried basil
- ✿ ¼ teaspoon dried parsley
- ✿ ¼ teaspoon red pepper flakes
- ✿ 1 cup water

1. Grease a baking pan with 2 teaspoons of the avocado oil.
2. Press the Sauté button on the Instant Pot and heat the remaining 1⅓ tablespoons of the avocado oil. Add the onion and bell peppers to the pot and sauté for 3 minutes, or until tender. Add the ham and continue to sauté for 2 minutes. Transfer the ham and onion mixture to a bowl. Clean the pot.
3. In a medium bowl, whisk together the eggs, cream, salt, black pepper, basil, parsley and pepper flakes. Pour the mixture into the prepared baking pan. Stir in the ham and onion mixture. Cover the pan with foil.
4. Pour the water and insert the trivet in the Instant Pot. Put the pan on the trivet.
5. Lock the lid. Select the Manual mode and set the cooking time for 35 minutes on High Pressure. Once the timer goes off, perform a natural pressure release for 10 minutes, then release any remaining pressure. Carefully open the lid.
6. Remove the baking pan from the pot. Serve hot.

Per Serving
calories: 571 | fat: 43.4g | protein: 39.1g | carbs: 6.0g | net carbs: 5.1g | fiber: 0.9g

Bacon and Broccoli Frittata

Prep time: 5 minutes | Cook time: 19 minutes | Serves 2

- ✿ 2 teaspoons avocado oil
- ✿ 4 slices bacon
- ✿ 2 cups chopped broccoli
- ✿ ½ teaspoon sea salt
- ✿ ¼ teaspoon ground black pepper
- ✿ 4 large eggs
- ✿ ¼ cup heavy whipping cream
- ✿ ¼ teaspoon ground cumin
- ✿ ¾ cup crumbled Feta cheese
- ✿ 1 cup water

1. Use the avocado oil to grease a baking dish that fits inside your Instant Pot.
2. Set the Instant Pot to Sauté mode. When hot, add the bacon and cook, flipping occasionally, until the bacon is crispy. Remove to a plate.
3. Add the broccoli to the pot and season with ¼ teaspoon of the salt and ⅛ teaspoon of the pepper. Sauté for 3 minutes, then transfer the broccoli to a small bowl.
4. In a medium bowl, lightly beat together the eggs, cream, cumin, and the remaining ¼ teaspoon salt and ⅛ teaspoon pepper. Crumble the bacon and stir it into the eggs, along with half the feta cheese. Pour the egg mixture into the prepared baking dish. Quickly stir in the broccoli. Sprinkle with the remaining feta cheese. Cover with a metal or silicone lid, or use foil.
5. Wipe out the Instant Pot if desired. Pour in the water and place the trivet inside. Arrange the sling over it so the two ends stick up like handles, then lower the baking dish onto the sling and the trivet.
6. Lock the lid. Select the Manual mode and set the cooking time for 16 minutes on High Pressure. Once the timer goes off, perform a natural pressure release for 5 minutes, then release any remaining pressure. Carefully open the lid.
7. Use the sling to carefully remove the hot baking dish. Serve hot or at room temperature.

Per Serving
calories: 605 | fat: 52.2g | protein: 28.7g | carbs: 5.4g | net carbs: 4.2g | fiber: 1.2g

Warm Breakfast Salad with Sardines

Prep time: 10 minutes | Cook time: 14 to 15 minutes | Serves 2

- ✿ 2 large eggs
- ✿ 1 cup water
- ✿ 1 tablespoon avocado oil
- ✿ 4 slices bacon, cut into small pieces
- ✿ 2 tablespoons minced shallots
- ✿ 1 tablespoon apple cider vinegar
- ✿ 1 (4.4-ounce / 125-g) can oil-packed sardines
- ✿ ¼ cup fresh parsley leaves
- ✿ 4 cups chopped romaine lettuce
- ✿ 2 cups baby spinach, torn into smaller pieces
- ✿ ¼ teaspoon ground black pepper
- ✿ 1 medium avocado, sliced

1. Pour the water into the Instant Pot. Place the trivet inside and place the eggs on top.
2. Set the lid in place. Select the Manual mode and set the cooking time for 10 minutes on High Pressure.
3. Meanwhile, prepare a bowl with ice water to cool the eggs.
4. When the timer goes off, do a quick pressure release. Carefully open the lid. Use tongs to transfer the eggs to the ice bath. When cool, peel and slice the eggs.
5. Carefully pour the water out of the Instant Pot and wipe it dry. Set the Instant Pot to Sauté mode and heat the avocado oil. Add the bacon and cook for 3 minutes. Add the shallots and cook until the bacon is crispy, another 1 to 2 minutes. Press Cancel.
6. Deglaze the pot with the vinegar, scraping the bottom with a wooden spoon to loosen any browned bits. Use a fork to break up the sardines and add them, along with their oil, to the pot. Stir in the parsley.
7. Place the lettuce, spinach, and pepper in the pot and mix well to coat the greens with the oil. Divide the mixture between two large serving bowls, scraping any remaining dressing from the pot.
8. Top each salad with half the sliced avocado and 1 sliced egg. Crack some black pepper over the top and serve immediately.

Per Serving

calories: 679 | fat: 55.1g | protein: 33.4g | carbs: 16.0g | net carbs: 6.0g | fiber: 10.0g

Sumptuous Breakfast Stuffed Mushrooms

Prep time: 10 minutes | Cook time: 15 to 16 minutes | Serves 2

- ✿ 12 large white mushrooms, washed, stems removed and reserved
- ✿ 1 tablespoon avocado oil
- ✿ ¼ teaspoon kosher salt
- ✿ ¼ teaspoon ground black pepper
- ✿ 1 tablespoon butter
- ✿ 6 ounces (170 g) bulk pork breakfast sausage
- ✿ 1 clove garlic, minced
- ✿ ¼ cup full-fat coconut milk
- ✿ 1 cup finely chopped Swiss chard
- ✿ 1 cup water

1. Finely chop the mushroom stems and set aside. Place the mushroom caps stemmed side down in a medium bowl and pour the avocado oil over them. Season with the salt and pepper. Toss gently to coat the mushrooms with oil without breaking them.
2. Set the Instant Pot to Sauté mode and melt the butter. When it is melted, crumble in the sausage and add the chopped mushroom stems. Sauté, stirring occasionally, until only a little pink remains in the pork, 3 to 4 minutes. Add the garlic and sauté until the pork is cooked through.
3. Deglaze the pot with the coconut milk, scraping the bottom with a wooden spoon to loosen any browned bits. Stir in the chopped chard and cook just until they are wilted.
4. Transfer the pork to a bowl. Taste and adjust the salt and pepper. Wipe or wash out the pot insert.
5. Stuff the pork mixture into the mushrooms. Place the mushrooms stem side up in two stackable stainless steel insert pans, 6 mushrooms per pan. Stack and secure the lid on the pans.
6. Pour the water into the Instant Pot and lower the stacked pans into the pot.
7. Set the lid in place. Select the Steam mode and set the cooking time for 12 minutes on High Pressure. When the timer goes off, do a quick pressure release. Carefully open the lid.
8. Transfer the pan from the pot. Open the insert pans and transfer the mushrooms to serving plates. Serve warm.

Per Serving
calories: 453 | fat: 40.8g | protein: 16.1g | carbs: 8.1g | net carbs: 6.3g | fiber: 1.8g

Classic Cinnamon Roll Coffee Cake

Prep time: 10 minutes | Cook time: 45 minutes | Serves 8

Cake:
- ✿ 2 cups almond flour
- ✿ 1 cup granulated erythritol
- ✿ 1 teaspoon baking powder
- ✿ Pinch of salt
- ✿ 2 eggs
- ✿ ½ cup sour cream
- ✿ 4 tablespoons butter, melted
- ✿ 2 teaspoons vanilla extract
- ✿ 2 tablespoons Swerve
- ✿ 1½ teaspoons ground cinnamon
- ✿ Cooking spray
- ✿ ½ cup water

Icing:
- ✿ 2 ounces (56 g) cream cheese, softened
- ✿ 1 cup powdered erythritol
- ✿ 1 tablespoon heavy cream
- ✿ ½ teaspoon vanilla extract

1. In the bowl of a stand mixer, combine the almond flour, granulated erythritol, baking powder and salt. Mix until no lumps remain. Add the eggs, sour cream, butter and vanilla to the mixer bowl and mix until well combined.
2. In a separate bowl, mix together the Swerve and cinnamon.
3. Spritz the baking pan with cooking spray. Pour in the cake batter and use a knife to make sure it is level around the pan. Sprinkle the cinnamon mixture on top. Cover the pan tightly with aluminum foil.
4. Pour the water and insert the trivet in the Instant Pot. Put the pan on the trivet.
5. Set the lid in place. Select the Manual mode and set the cooking time for 45 minutes on High Pressure. When the timer goes off, do a quick pressure release. Carefully open the lid.
6. Remove the cake from the pot and remove the foil. Blot off any moisture on top of the cake with a paper towel, if necessary. Let rest in the pan for 5 minutes.
7. Meanwhile, make the icing: In a small bowl, use a mixer to whip the cream cheese until it is light and fluffy. Slowly fold in the powdered erythritol and mix until well combined. Add the heavy cream and vanilla extract and mix until thoroughly combined.
8. When the cake is cooled, transfer it to a platter and drizzle the icing all over.

Per Serving
calories: 313 | fat: 27.0g | protein: 8.7g | carbs: 6.8g | net carbs: 3.5g | fiber: 3.3g

Streusel Pumpkin Cake

Prep time: 10 minutes | Cook time: 30 minutes | Serves 8

Streusel Topping:
- ¼ cup Swerve
- ¼ cup almond flour
- 2 tablespoons coconut oil or unsalted butter, softened
- ½ teaspoon ground cinnamon

Cake:
- 2 large eggs, beaten
- 2 cups almond flour
- 1 cup pumpkin purée
- ¾ cup Swerve
- 2 teaspoons pumpkin pie spice
- 2 teaspoons vanilla extract
- ½ teaspoon fine sea salt

Glaze:
- ½ cup Swerve
- 3 tablespoons unsweetened almond milk

1. Set a trivet in the Instant Pot and pour in 1 cup water. Line a baking pan with parchment paper.
2. In a small bowl, whisk together all the ingredients for the streusel topping with a fork.
3. In a medium-sized bowl, stir together all the ingredients for the cake until thoroughly combined.
4. Scoop half of the batter into the prepared baking pan and sprinkle half of the streusel topping on top. Repeat with the remaining batter and topping.
5. Place the baking pan on the trivet in the Instant Pot.
6. Lock the lid, select the Manual mode and set the cooking time for 30 minutes on High Pressure.
7. Meanwhile, whisk together the Swerve and almond milk in a small bowl until it reaches a runny consistency.
8. When the timer goes off, do a natural pressure release for 10 minutes, then release any remaining pressure. Open the lid.
9. Remove the baking pan from the pot. Let cool in the pan for 10 minutes. Transfer the cake onto a plate and peel off the parchment paper.
10. Transfer the cake onto a serving platter. Spoon the glaze over the top of the cake. Serve immediately.

Per Serving
calories: 238 | fat: 20g | protein: 9.1g | carbs: 9.0g | net carbs: 4.9g | fiber: 4.1g

Bacon and Spinach Eggs

Prep time: 5 minutes | Cook time: 9 minutes | Serves 4

- ✿ 2 tablespoons unsalted butter, divided
- ✿ ½ cup diced bacon
- ✿ ⅓ cup finely diced shallots
- ✿ ⅓ cup chopped spinach, leaves only
- ✿ Pinch of sea salt
- ✿ Pinch of black pepper
- ✿ ½ cup water
- ✿ ¼ cup heavy whipping cream
- ✿ 8 large eggs
- ✿ 1 tablespoon chopped fresh chives, for garnish

1. Set the Instant Pot on the Sauté mode and melt 1 tablespoon of the butter. Add the bacon to the pot and sauté for about 4 minutes, or until crispy. Using a slotted spoon, transfer the bacon bits to a bowl and set aside.
2. Add the remaining 1 tablespoon of the butter and shallots to the pot and sauté for about 2 minutes, or until tender. Add the spinach leaves and sauté for 1 minute, or until wilted. Season with sea salt and black pepper and stir. Transfer the spinach to a separate bowl and set aside.
3. Drain the oil from the pot into a bowl. Pour in the water and put the trivet inside.
4. With a paper towel, coat four ramekins with the bacon grease. In each ramekin, place 1 tablespoon of the heavy whipping cream, reserved bacon bits and sautéed spinach. Crack two eggs without breaking the yolks in each ramekin. Cover the ramekins with aluminum foil. Place two ramekins on the trivet and stack the other two on top.
5. Lock the lid. Select the Manual mode and set the cooking time for 2 minutes at Low Pressure. When the timer goes off, use a natural pressure release for 5 minutes, then release any remaining pressure. Carefully open the lid.
6. Carefully take out the ramekins and serve garnished with the chives.

Per Serving
calories: 320 | fat: 25.8g | protein: 17.2g | carbs: 4.0g | net carbs: 3.9g | fiber: 0.1g

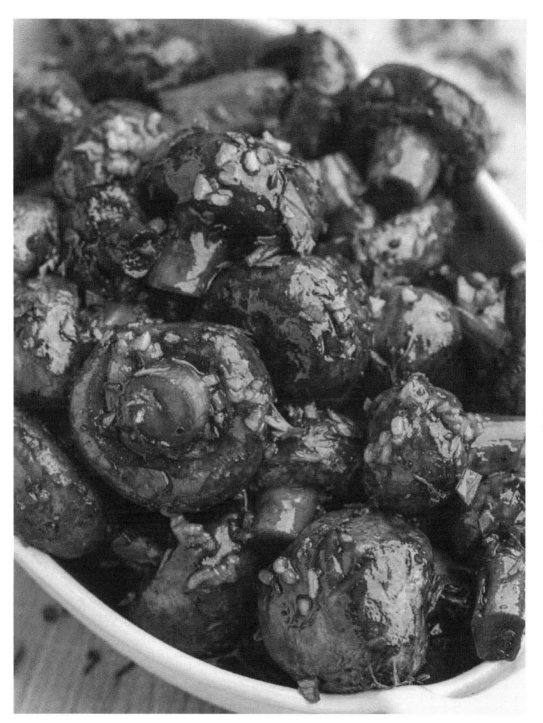

Appetizers and Sides

Herbed Mushrooms

Prep time: 5 minutes | Cook time: 10 minutes | Serves 4

- ✿ 2 tablespoons butter
- ✿ 2 cloves garlic, minced
- ✿ 20 ounces (567 g) button mushrooms
- ✿ 1 tablespoon coconut aminos
- ✿ 1 teaspoon dried rosemary
- ✿ 1 teaspoon dried basil
- ✿ 1 teaspoon dried sage
- ✿ 1 bay leaf
- ✿ Sea salt, to taste
- ✿ ½ teaspoon freshly ground black pepper
- ✿ ½ cup chicken broth
- ✿ ½ cup water
- ✿ 1 tablespoon roughly chopped fresh parsley leaves, for garnish

1. Set your Instant Pot to Sauté and melt the butter.
2. Add the garlic and mushrooms and sauté for 3 to 4 minutes until the garlic is fragrant.
3. Add the remaining ingredients except the parsley to the Instant Pot and stir well.
4. Lock the lid. Select the Manual mode and set the cooking time for 5 minutes at High Pressure.
5. When the timer beeps, perform a quick pressure release. Carefully open the lid.
6. Remove the mushrooms from the pot to a platter. Serve garnished with the fresh parsley leaves.

Per Serving

calories: 94 | fat: 6.8g | protein: 5.7g | carbs: 5.3g | net carbs: 3.6g | fiber: 1.7g

Stuffed Jalapeños with Bacon

Prep time: 10 minutes | Cook time: 6 minutes | Serves 2

- ✿ 1 ounce (28 g) bacon, chopped, fried
- ✿ 2 ounces (57 g) Cheddar cheese, shredded
- ✿ 1 tablespoon coconut cream
- ✿ 1 teaspoon chopped green onions
- ✿ 2 jalapeños, trimmed and seeded

1. Mix together the chopped bacon, cheese, coconut cream, and green onions in a mixing bowl and stir until well incorporated.
2. Stuff the jalapeños evenly with the bacon mixture.
3. Press the Sauté button to heat your Instant Pot.
4. Place the stuffed jalapeños in the Instant Pot and cook each side for 3 minutes until softened.
5. Transfer to a paper towel-lined plate and serve.

Per Serving

calories: 216 | fat: 17.5g | protein: 12.9g | carbs: 1.7g | net carbs: 1.1g | fiber: 0.6g

Cauliflower Cheese Balls

Prep time: 5 minutes | Cook time: 21 minutes | Serves 8

- ❁ 1 cup water
- ❁ 1 head cauliflower, broken into florets
- ❁ 1 cup shredded Asiago cheese
- ❁ ½ cup grated Parmesan cheese
- ❁ 2 eggs, beaten
- ❁ 2 tablespoons butter
- ❁ 2 tablespoons minced fresh chives
- ❁ 1 garlic clove, minced
- ❁ ½ teaspoon cayenne pepper
- ❁ Coarse sea salt and white pepper, to taste

1. Pour the water into the Instant Pot and insert a steamer basket. Place the cauliflower in the basket.
2. Lock the lid. Select the Manual mode and set the cooking time for 3 minutes at High Pressure.
3. When the timer beeps, perform a quick pressure release. Carefully remove the lid.
4. Transfer the cauliflower to a food processor, along with the remaining ingredients. Pulse until everything is well combined.
5. Form the mixture into bite-sized balls and place them on a baking sheet.
6. Bake in the preheated oven at 400ºF (205ºC) for 18 minutes until golden brown. Flip the balls halfway through the cooking time.
7. Cool for 5 minutes before serving.

Per Serving

calories: 161 | fat: 12.6g | protein: 9.3g | carbs: 3.8g | net carbs: 3g | fiber: 0.8g

Cheesy Zucchini Rings

Prep time: 15 minutes | Cook time: 3 minutes | Serves 2

- ❁ 1 zucchini
- ❁ 2 teaspoon butter, softened
- ❁ 1 cup shredded Cheddar cheese
- ❁ 2 cup water

1. Slice the zucchini into rings and remove the center of every ring.
2. Coat a baking pan with the softened butter and place the zucchini rings in a single layer. Fill each ring with the shredded cheese.
3. Pour the water into the Instant Pot and insert the trivet. Place the baking pan with zucchini rings on the trivet.
4. Secure the lid. Select the Manual mode and set the cooking time for 3 minutes at High Pressure.
5. Once cooking is complete, do a quick pressure release. Carefully open the lid.
6. Let the zucchini rings cool for 5 minutes and serve.

Per Serving

calories: 279 | fat: 22.9g | protein: 15.5g | carbs: 3.9g | net carbs: 2.7g | fiber: 1.2g

Cheesy Cauliflower Tots

Prep time: 5 minutes | Cook time: 20 minutes | Serves 6

- ✿ 1 cup water
- ✿ 1 head cauliflower, broken into florets
- ✿ 2 eggs, beaten
- ✿ 2 tablespoons chopped fresh coriander

- ✿ 1 shallot, peeled and chopped
- ✿ ½ cup grated Parmesan cheese
- ✿ ½ cup grated Swiss cheese
- ✿ Sea salt and ground black pepper, to taste

1. Pour the water into the Instant Pot and insert a steamer basket. Place the cauliflower florets in the basket.
2. Lock the lid. Select the Manual mode and set the cooking time for 3 minutes at High Pressure.
3. When the timer beeps, perform a quick pressure release. Carefully remove the lid.
4. Transfer the cauliflower to a food processor, along with the remaining ingredients. Pulse until everything is well incorporated.
5. Form the mixture into a tater-tot shape with oiled hands. Arrange the cauliflower tots on a lightly greased baking sheet.
6. Bake in the preheated oven at 400ºF (205ºC) for 15 to 18 minutes. Flip them halfway through the cooking time.
7. Remove from the oven to a plate and serve.

Per Serving
calories: 137 | fat: 8.9g | protein: 9.6g | carbs: 4.3g | net carbs: 3.2g | fiber: 1.1g

Lemon Brussels Sprouts

Prep time: 5 minutes | Cook time: 5 minutes | Serves 4

- ✿ 2 tablespoons extra-virgin olive oil
- ✿ 1 pound (454 g) Brussels sprouts, outer leaves removed, and washed
- ✿ 1 lemon, juiced

- ✿ ½ teaspoon fresh paprika
- ✿ ½ teaspoon kosher salt
- ✿ ½ teaspoon black ground pepper
- ✿ 1 cup bone broth

1. Set your Instant Pot to Sauté and heat the olive oil.
2. Add the remaining ingredients except the bone broth to the Instant Pot and cook for 1 minute. Pour in the broth.
3. Secure the lid. Select the Manual mode and set the cooking time for 3 minutes at Low Pressure.
4. Once cooking is complete, do a quick pressure release. Carefully open the lid.
5. Remove the Brussels sprouts from the Instant Pot to a plate and serve.

Per Serving
calories: 124 | fat: 7.7g | protein: 5.6g | carbs: 12.2g | net carbs: 7.4g | fiber: 4.8g

Easy Deviled Eggs

Prep time: 5 minutes | Cook time: 5 minutes | Serves 8

- 1 cup water
- 8 eggs
- ½ can tuna in spring water, drained
- ¼ cup mayonnaise
- 2 tablespoons finely chopped spring

- onions
- 1 teaspoon Dijon mustard
- 1 teaspoon cayenne pepper
- ⅓ teaspoon fresh or dried dill weed
- Salt and white pepper, to taste

1. Pour the water into the Instant Pot and insert a steamer basket. Place the eggs in the basket.
2. Lock the lid. Select the Manual mode and set the cooking time for 5 minutes at Low Pressure.
3. When the timer beeps, perform a quick pressure release. Carefully remove the lid.
4. Let the eggs cool for 10 to 15 minutes. When cooled, peel the eggs and slice them into halves. Scoop the egg yolks into a small bowl and add the remaining ingredients. Using a fork, mash until blended.
5. Spoon 1 to 2 teaspoons of the egg yolk mixture into each egg white half. Serve chilled.

Per Serving

calories: 161 | fat: 11.7g | protein: 11.1g | carbs: 3.0g | net carbs: 2.7g | fiber: 0.3g

Parsley Fennel Slices

Prep time: 10 minutes | Cook time: 5 minutes | Serves 2

- 1 cup water
- 1 fennel bulb, sliced
- ¾ cup chopped fresh parsley

- 1 tablespoon olive oil
- 1 tablespoon coconut aminos
- 1 teaspoon apple cider vinegar

1. Pour the water into the Instant Pot and insert a steamer basket. Place the sliced fennel in the basket.
2. Secure the lid. Select the Steam mode and set the cooking time for 5 minutes at High Pressure.
3. Once cooking is complete, do a quick pressure release. Carefully open the lid.
4. Remove the fennel from the Instant Pot to a bowl. Add the remaining ingredients to the bowl and gently toss until combined. Serve immediately.

Per Serving

calories: 115 | fat: 7.6g | protein: 2.4g | carbs: 11.4g | net carbs: 7.0g | fiber: 4.4g

Salmon Salad with Feta Cheese

Prep time: 10 minutes | Cook time: 4 minutes | Serves 2

- 6 ounces (170 g) salmon
- ½ teaspoon salt
- 1 cup water
- 1 cup chopped lettuce
- 1 teaspoon olive oil
- 2 ounces (57 g) feta cheese, crumbled

1. Season the salmon with salt and wrap in foil.
2. Pour the water into the Instant Pot and insert the trivet. Place the salmon on the trivet.
3. Secure the lid. Select the Manual mode and set the cooking time for 4 minutes at High Pressure.
4. Meanwhile, toss the lettuce with the olive oil in a salad bowl.
5. When the timer beeps, perform a quick pressure release. Carefully remove the lid.
6. Remove the salmon and chop it roughly, then transfer to the salad bowl. Sprinkle with the feta cheese and gently toss to combine. Serve immediately.

Per Serving

calories: 213 | fat: 13.9g | protein: 20.9g | carbs: 1.9g | net carbs: 1.7g | fiber: 0.2g

Pepperoni Pizza Bites

Prep time: 5 minutes | Cook time: 5 minutes | Serves 4 to 5

- 1 cup water
- 2 cups shredded full-fat mozzarella cheese
- 1 cup grated full-fat Parmesan cheese
- 1 (14-ounce / 397-g) can sugar-free diced

- tomatoes, drained
- 16 uncured pepperoni slices, cut in half
- 1 teaspoon dried oregano
- 1 teaspoon dried basil

1. Pour the water into the Instant Pot and insert the trivet.
2. Combine the remaining ingredients in a large bowl and stir to incorporate.
3. Spoon the mixture into a greased egg bites mold. Work in batches, if needed. I prefer to stack 2 egg bites molds on top of each other, separated by Mason jar lids. Put the molds on the trivet and loosely cover with aluminum foil.
4. Secure the lid. Select the Manual mode and set the cooking time for 5 minutes at High Pressure.
5. Once cooking is complete, do a natural pressure release for 10 minutes, then release any remaining pressure. Carefully open the lid.
6. Remove the molds and cool for 5 minutes, then serve.

Per Serving

calories: 331 | fat: 25.1g | protein: 22.5g | carbs: 6.3g | net carbs: 4.6g | fiber: 1.7g

Herbed Shrimp

Prep time: 5 minutes | Cook time: 5 minutes | Serves 4

- 2 tablespoons olive oil
- ¾ pound (340 g) shrimp, peeled and deveined
- 1 teaspoon paprika
- 1 teaspoon garlic powder
- 1 teaspoon onion powder
- 1 teaspoon dried parsley flakes
- ½ teaspoon dried oregano
- ½ teaspoon dried thyme
- ½ teaspoon dried basil
- ½ teaspoon dried rosemary
- ¼ teaspoon red pepper flakes
- Coarse sea salt and ground black pepper, to taste
- 1 cup chicken broth

1. Set your Instant Pot to Sauté and heat the olive oil.
2. Add the shrimp and sauté for 2 to 3 minutes.
3. Add the remaining ingredients to the Instant Pot and stir to combine.
4. Secure the lid. Select the Manual mode and set the cooking time for 2 minutes at Low Pressure.
5. When the timer beeps, perform a quick pressure release. Carefully remove the lid.
6. Transfer the shrimp to a plate and serve.

Per Serving
calories: 146 | fat: 7.7g | protein: 18.5g | carbs: 3.0g | net carbs: 2.3g | fiber: 0.7g

Paprika Egg Salad

Prep time: 5 minutes | Cook time: 7 minutes | Serves 2

- 6 eggs
- 1 cup water
- ¼ cup mayonnaise
- ½ teaspoon ground turmeric
- ½ teaspoon fresh paprika
- ½ teaspoon kosher salt
- ½ teaspoon freshly ground black pepper
- ¼ cup thinly sliced green onions

1. Beat the eggs in a bowl until frothy.
2. Pour the water into the Instant Pot and insert the trivet. Place the bowl with the eggs on the trivet.
3. Secure the lid. Select the Manual mode and set the cooking time for 7 minutes at High Pressure.
4. Meanwhile, stir together the mayo, turmeric, paprika, salt, and pepper in a small bowl until well combined.
5. When the timer beeps, perform a natural pressure release for 10 minutes, then release any remaining pressure. Carefully open the lid.
6. Remove the eggs and allow to cool for a few minutes. Stir in the mayo mixture and serve topped with the green onions.

Per Serving
calories: 400 | fat: 37.6g | protein: 17.5g | carbs: 3.0g | net carbs: 2.2g | fiber: 0.8g

Chinese Spare Ribs

Prep time: 3 minutes | Cook time: 24 minutes | Serves 6

- 1½ pounds (680 g) spare ribs
- Salt and ground black pepper, to taste
- 2 tablespoons sesame oil
- ½ cup chopped green onions
- ½ cup chicken stock
- 2 tomatoes, crushed
- 2 tablespoons sherry
- 1 tablespoon coconut aminos
- 1 teaspoon ginger-garlic paste
- ½ teaspoon crushed red pepper flakes
- ½ teaspoon dried parsley
- 2 tablespoons sesame seeds, for serving

1. Season the spare ribs with salt and black pepper to taste.
2. Set your Instant Pot to Sauté and heat the sesame oil.
3. Add the seasoned spare ribs and sear each side for about 3 minutes.
4. Add the remaining ingredients except the sesame seeds to the Instant Pot and stir well.
5. Secure the lid. Select the Meat/Stew mode and set the cooking time for 18 minutes at High Pressure.
6. When the timer beeps, perform a natural pressure release for 10 minutes, then release any remaining pressure. Carefully remove the lid.
7. Serve topped with the sesame seeds.

Per Serving

calories: 336 | fat: 16.3g | protein: 42.6g | carbs: 3.0g | net carbs: 2.0g | fiber: 1.0g

Bok Choy Salad Boats with Shrimp

Prep time: 8 minutes | Cook time: 2 minutes | Serves 8

- 26 shrimp, cleaned and deveined
- 2 tablespoons fresh lemon juice
- 1 cup water
- Sea salt and ground black pepper, to taste
- 4 ounces (113 g) feta cheese, crumbled
- 2 tomatoes, diced
- ⅓ cup olives, pitted and sliced
- 4 tablespoons olive oil
- 2 tablespoons apple cider vinegar
- 8 Bok choy leaves
- 2 tablespoons fresh basil leaves, snipped
- 2 tablespoons chopped fresh mint leaves

1. Toss the shrimp and lemon juice in the Instant Pot until well coated. Pour in the water.
2. Lock the lid. Select the Manual mode and set the cooking time for 2 minutes at Low Pressure.
3. When the timer beeps, perform a quick pressure release. Carefully remove the lid.
4. Season the shrimp with salt and pepper to taste, then let them cool completely.
5. Toss the shrimp with the feta cheese, tomatoes, olives, olive oil, and vinegar until well incorporated.
6. Divide the salad evenly onto each Bok choy leaf and place them on a serving plate. Scatter the basil and mint leaves on top and serve immediately.

Per Serving

calories: 129 | fat: 10.7g | protein: 4.9g | carbs: 3.0g | net carbs: 2.4g | fiber: 0.6g

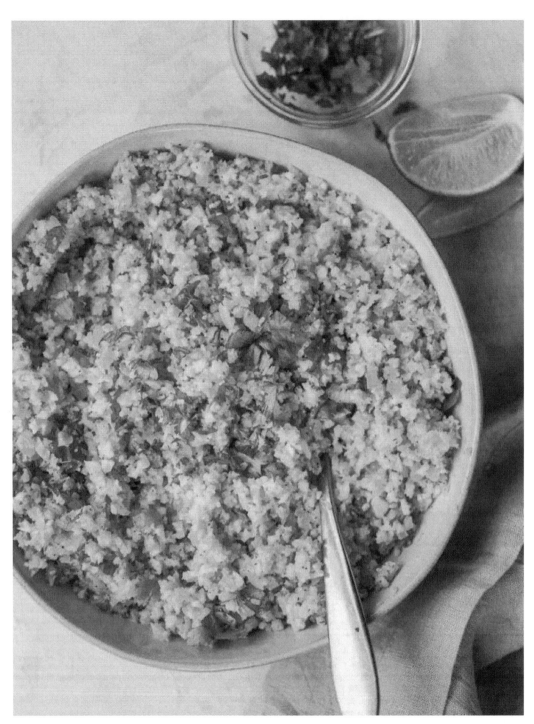

CHAPTER 5
Vegetables

Lime Cauliflower Rice with Cilantro

Prep time: 5 minutes | Cook time: 8 minutes | Serves 4

- ✿ 1 head cauliflower, trimmed, stem removed and cut into medium florets
- ✿ 1 cup water
- ✿ 2 tablespoons avocado oil
- ✿ 1 garlic clove, minced
- ✿ Juice of 1 lime
- ✿ ⅛ teaspoon fine grind sea salt
- ✿ 4 sprigs fresh cilantro, chopped

1. Pour the water into the Instant Pot and put the trivet in the pot. Place the cauliflower florets in the trivet. Place a steamer basket on the trivet. Add the cauliflower to the steamer basket.
2. Lock the lid. Select the Manual mode and set the cooking time for 2 minutes on High Pressure. When the timer goes off, perform a quick pressure release. Carefully open the lid.
3. Remove the steamer basket and cauliflower from the pot. Place the cauliflower florets in a blender and pulse until it reaches a rice-like texture. Set aside.
4. Pour out the water and wipe the pot dry with a paper towel.
5. Select Sauté mode and heat the avocado oil. Add the garlic to the pot and sauté for 2 minutes, or until fragrant.
6. Add the cauliflower rice to the pot and sauté for 2 additional minutes, or until the rice becomes soft. Stir in the lime juice and sauté for 2 additional minutes.
7. Transfer the cauliflower rice to a serving dish. Season with the sea salt and garnish with the cilantro. Serve hot.

Per Serving

calories: 106 | fat: 7.1g | protein: 3.1g | carbs: 7.4g | net carbs: 4.0g | fiber: 3.4g

Savory and Rich Creamed Kale

Prep time: 10 minutes | Cook time: 5 minutes | Serves 4

- ✿ 2 tablespoons extra-virgin olive oil
- ✿ 2 cloves garlic, crushed
- ✿ 1 small onion, chopped
- ✿ 12 ounces (340 g) kale, finely chopped
- ✿ ½ cup chicken broth
- ✿ 1 teaspoon Herbes de Provence
- ✿ 4 ounces (113 g) cream cheese
- ✿ ½ cup full-fat heavy cream
- ✿ 1 teaspoon dried tarragon

1. Press the Sauté button on the Instant Pot and heat the olive oil. Add the garlic and onion to the pot and sauté for 2 minutes, or until the onion is soft. Stir in the kale, chicken broth and Herbes de Provence.
2. Lock the lid. Select the Manual mode and set the cooking time for 3 minutes at High Pressure. When the timer goes off, perform a quick pressure release. Carefully open the lid.
3. Stir in the cream cheese, heavy cream and tarragon. Stir well to thicken the dish. Serve immediately.

Per Serving

calories: 229 | fat: 19.0g | protein: 6.1g | carbs: 11.9g | net carbs: 8.5g | fiber: 3.4g

Broiled Cauli Bites

Prep time: 10 minutes | Cook time: 1 to 2 minutes | Serves 4

- ✿ 1 head cauliflower, cut into florets
- ✿ 1 cup water
- ✿ 1 cup mayonnaise
- ✿ ⅓ cup full-fat coconut milk yogurt
- ✿ 1 teaspoon dried dill
- ✿ 1 teaspoon onion powder
- ✿ 1 teaspoon garlic powder
- ✿ ½ teaspoon sea salt
- ✿ 1 teaspoon apple cider vinegar
- ✿ 4 tablespoons melted butter, divided
- ✿ 3 tablespoons hot sauce
- ✿ 2 celery stalks, cut into 3-inch pieces

1. Pour the water into the Instant Pot and put the steamer basket in the pot. Place the cauliflower florets in the steamer basket.
2. Close and secure the lid. Select the Manual mode and set the cooking time for 0 minute at High Pressure.
3. Meanwhile, stir together the mayonnaise, coconut milk yogurt, dill, onion powder, garlic powder, sea salt and apple cider vinegar in a bowl. Set in a refrigerator. In another bowl, whisk together the melted butter and hot sauce.
4. Preheat the oven to 450°F (235°C).
5. When the timer beeps, use a quick pressure release. Carefully open the lid.
6. Transfer the florets to a large mixing bowl and coat the florets well with the butter and hot sauce mixture.
7. Spread the coated florets on a baking pan and place the pan in the oven. Broil for 1 to 2 minutes, or until the florets are browned.
8. Remove the mayonnaise mixture from the refrigerator. Serve the Buffalo Cauli Bites and celery sticks with the mayonnaise mixture.

Per Serving
calories: 546 | fat: 57.8g | protein: 2.8g | carbs: 6.2g | net carbs: 4.0g | fiber: 2.2g

Satarash with Eggs

Prep time: 10 minutes | Cook time: 5 minutes | Serves 4

- ✿ 2 tablespoons olive oil
- ✿ 1 white onion, chopped
- ✿ 2 cloves garlic
- ✿ 2 ripe tomatoes, puréed
- ✿ 1 green bell pepper, deseeded and sliced
- ✿ 1 red bell pepper, deseeded and sliced
- ✿ 1 teaspoon paprika
- ✿ ½ teaspoon dried oregano
- ✿ ½ teaspoon turmeric
- ✿ Kosher salt and ground black pepper, to taste
- ✿ 1 cup water
- ✿ 4 large eggs, lightly whisked

1. Press the Sauté button on the Instant Pot and heat the olive oil. Add the onion and garlic to the pot and sauté for 2 minutes, or until fragrant. Stir in the remaining ingredients, except for the eggs.
2. Lock the lid. Select the Manual mode and set the cooking time for 3 minutes on High Pressure. When the timer goes off, perform a quick pressure release. Carefully open the lid.
3. Fold in the eggs and stir to combine. Lock the lid and let it sit in the residual heat for 5 minutes. Serve warm.

Per Serving
calories: 169 | fat: 11.9g | protein: 7.8g | carbs: 8.9g | net carbs: 6.8g | fiber: 2.1g

Chanterelle Mushrooms with Cheddar Cheese

Prep time: 10 minutes | Cook time: 5 minutes | Serves 4

- 1 tablespoon olive oil
- 2 cloves garlic, minced
- 1 (1-inch) ginger root, grated
- 16 ounces (454 g) Chanterelle mushrooms, brushed clean and sliced
- ½ cup unsweetened tomato purée
- ½ cup water
- 2 tablespoons dry white wine
- 1 teaspoon dried basil
- ½ teaspoon dried thyme
- ½ teaspoon dried dill weed
- ⅓ teaspoon freshly ground black pepper
- Kosher salt, to taste
- 1 cup shredded Cheddar cheese

1. Press the Sauté button on the Instant Pot and heat the olive oil. Add the garlic and grated ginger to the pot and sauté for 1 minute, or until fragrant. Stir in the remaining ingredients, except for the cheese.
2. Lock the lid. Select the Manual mode and set the cooking time for 5 minutes on Low Pressure. When the timer goes off, perform a quick pressure release. Carefully open the lid..
3. Serve topped with the shredded cheese.

Per Serving

calories: 206 | fat: 13.7g | protein: 9.3g | carbs: 12.3g | net carbs: 7.1g | fiber: 5.2g

Cheesy Cauliflower Flatbread

Prep time: 10 minutes | Cook time: 2 hours 30 minutes | Serves 8

- ½ medium head cauliflower, trimmed, stem removed and cut into florets
- 3½ tablespoons coconut flour
- 1½ cups grated Mouncezarella cheese, divided
- ¼ teaspoon fine grind sea salt
- 2 large eggs, beaten
- 2 tablespoons heavy cream
- 2 tablespoons unsalted butter, melted, divided
- 2 garlic cloves, minced
- 2 tablespoons fresh basil, cut into ribbons

1. Add the cauliflower to a blender and pulse until it reaches a rice-like texture.
2. In a large bowl, whisk together ⅔ cup of the riced cauliflower, coconut flour, ¾ cup of the Mouncezarella cheese and sea salt. Stir in the eggs, heavy cream and 1 tablespoon of the butter.
3. Brush the Instant Pot with the remaining 1 tablespoon of the butter. Add the cauliflower mixture and use a spoon to press the mixture flat into the bottom of the pot. Sprinkle the garlic and the remaining ¾ cup of the Mouncezarella cheese on top.
4. Lock the lid. Select the Slow Cook mode and set the cooking time for 2 hours 30 minutes on More.
5. While the flatbread is cooking, preheat the oven broiler to 450ºF (235ºC).
6. Once the cook time is complete, transfer the flatbread to a clean work surface and cut into 8 wedges. Place the wedges on a large baking sheet and transfer to the oven to broil for 2 to 3 minutes, or until the cheese is lightly browned.
7. Remove from the oven and transfer to a serving platter. Sprinkle the basil ribbons on top. Serve warm.

Per Serving

calories: 136 | fat: 10.1g | protein: 6.2g | carbs: 5.3g | net carbs: 2.0g | fiber: 3.3g

Spaghetti Squash Noodles with Tomatoes

Prep time: 15 minutes | Cook time: 14 to 16 minutes | Serves 4

- 1 medium spaghetti squash
- 1 cup water
- 2 tablespoons olive oil
- 1 small yellow onion, diced
- 6 garlic cloves, minced
- 2 teaspoons crushed red pepper flakes
- 2 teaspoons dried oregano
- 1 cup sliced cherry tomatoes
- 1 teaspoon kosher salt
- ½ teaspoon freshly ground black pepper
- 1 (14.5-ounce / 411-g) can sugar-free crushed tomatoes
- ¼ cup capers
- 1 tablespoon caper brine
- ½ cup sliced olives

1. With a sharp knife, halve the spaghetti squash crosswise. Using a spoon, scoop out the seeds and sticky gunk in the middle of each half.
2. Pour the water into the Instant Pot and place the trivet in the pot with the handles facing up. Arrange the squash halves, cut side facing up, on the trivet.
3. Lock the lid. Select the Manual mode and set the cooking time for 7 minutes on High Pressure. When the timer goes off, use a quick pressure release. Carefully open the lid.
4. Remove the trivet and pour out the water that has collected in the squash cavities. Using the tines of a fork, separate the cooked strands into spaghetti-like pieces and set aside in a bowl.
5. Pour the water out of the pot. Select the Sauté mode and heat the oil.
6. Add the onion to the pot and sauté for 3 minutes. Add the garlic, pepper flakes and oregano to the pot and sauté for 1 minute.
7. Stir in the cherry tomatoes, salt and black pepper and cook for 2 minutes, or until the tomatoes are tender.
8. Pour in the crushed tomatoes, capers, caper brine and olives and bring the mixture to a boil. Continue to cook for 2 to 3 minutes to allow the flavors to meld.
9. Stir in the spaghetti squash noodles and cook for 1 to 2 minutes to warm everything through.
10. Transfer the dish to a serving platter and serve.

Per Serving
calories: 132 | fat: 9.3g | protein: 2.9g | carbs: 12.7g | net carbs: 7.8g | fiber: 4.9g

Green Beans with Onion

Prep time: 5 minutes | Cook time: 6 to 7 minutes | Serves 6

- 6 slices bacon, diced
- 1 cup diced onion
- 4 cups halved green beans
- ¼ cup water
- 1 teaspoon salt
- 1 teaspoon freshly ground black pepper

1. Press the Sauté button on the Instant Pot and add the bacon and onion to the pot and sauté for 2 to 3 minutes. Stir in the remaining ingredients.
2. Close and secure the lid. Select the Manual setting and set the cooking time for 4 minutes at High Pressure. Once the timer goes off, use a quick pressure release. Carefully open the lid.
3. Serve immediately.

Per Serving
calories: 166 | fat: 13.1g | protein: 6.2g | carbs: 5.8g | net carbs: 3.0g | fiber: 2.8g

Lemony Asparagus with Gremolata

Prep time: 15 minutes | Cook time: 2 minutes | Serves 2 to 4

Gremolata:
- 1 cup finely chopped fresh Italian flat-leaf parsley leaves

Asparagus:
- 1½ pounds (680 g) asparagus, trimmed
- 1 cup water
- Lemony Vinaigrette:
- 1½ tablespoons fresh lemon juice
- 1 teaspoon Swerve

Garnish:
- 3 tablespoons slivered almonds

- 3 garlic cloves, peeled and grated
- Zest of 2 small lemons

- 1 teaspoon Dijon mustard
- 2 tablespoons extra-virgin olive oil
- Kosher salt and freshly ground black pepper, to taste

1. In a small bowl, stir together all the ingredients for the gremolata.
2. Pour the water into the Instant Pot. Arrange the asparagus in a steamer basket. Lower the steamer basket into the pot.
3. Lock the lid. Select the Steam mode and set the cooking time for 2 minutes on Low Pressure.
4. Meanwhile, prepare the lemony vinaigrette: In a bowl, combine the lemon juice, swerve and mustard and whisk to combine. Slowly drizzle in the olive oil and continue to whisk. Season generously with salt and pepper.
5. When the timer goes off, perform a quick pressure release. Carefully open the lid. Remove the steamer basket from the Instant Pot.
6. Transfer the asparagus to a serving platter. Drizzle with the vinaigrette and sprinkle with the gremolata. Serve the asparagus topped with the slivered almonds.

Per Serving

calories: 277 | fat: 18.8g | protein: 10.9g | carbs: 23.8g | net carbs: 13.4g | fiber: 10.4g

Falafel and Lettuce Salad

Prep time: 10 minutes | Cook time: 6 to 8 minutes | Serves 4

- 1 cup shredded cauliflower
- ⅓ cup coconut flour
- 1 teaspoon grated lemon zest
- 1 egg, beaten
- 2 tablespoons coconut oil

- 2 cups chopped lettuce
- 1 cucumber, chopped
- 1 tablespoon olive oil
- 1 teaspoon lemon juice
- ½ teaspoon cayenne pepper

1. In a bowl, combine the cauliflower, coconut flour, grated lemon zest and egg. Form the mixture into small balls.
2. Set the Instant Pot to the Sauté mode and melt the coconut oil. Place the balls in the pot in a single layer. Cook for 3 to 4 minutes per side, or until they are golden brown.
3. In a separate bowl, stir together the remaining ingredients.
4. Place the cooked balls on top and serve.

Per Serving

calories: 175 | fat: 13.4g | protein: 4.7g | carbs: 11.1g | net carbs: 5.9g | fiber: 5.2g

Garlicky Broccoli with Roasted Almonds

Prep time: 10 minutes | Cook time: 4 minutes | Serves 4 to 6

- ✿ 6 cups broccoli florets
- ✿ 1 cup water
- ✿ 1½ tablespoons olive oil
- ✿ 8 garlic cloves, thinly sliced
- ✿ 2 shallots, thinly sliced
- ✿ ½ teaspoon crushed red pepper flakes
- ✿ Grated zest and juice of 1 medium lemon
- ✿ ½ teaspoon kosher salt
- ✿ Freshly ground black pepper, to taste
- ✿ ¼ cup chopped roasted almonds
- ✿ ¼ cup finely slivered fresh basil

1. Pour the water into the Instant Pot. Place the broccoli florets in a steamer basket and lower into the pot.
2. Close and secure the lid. Select the Steam setting and set the cooking time for 2 minutes at Low Pressure. Once the timer goes off, use a quick pressure release. Carefully open the lid.
3. Transfer the broccoli to a large bowl filled with cold water and ice. Once cooled, drain the broccoli and pat dry.
4. Select the Sauté mode on the Instant Pot and heat the olive oil. Add the garlic to the pot and sauté for 30 seconds, tossing constantly. Add the shallots and pepper flakes to the pot and sauté for 1 minute.
5. Stir in the cooked broccoli, lemon juice, salt and black pepper. Toss the ingredients together and cook for 1 minute.
6. Transfer the broccoli to a serving platter and sprinkle with the chopped almonds, lemon zest and basil. Serve immediately.

Per Serving
calories: 127 | fat: 8.2g | protein: 5.1g | carbs: 12.2g | net carbs: 10.6g | fiber: 1.6g

Smoked Paprika Cauliflower Balls

Prep time: 10 minutes | Cook time: 2 minutes | Serves 8

- ✿ 1 pound (454 g) cauliflower, cut into florets
- ✿ 1 cup water
- ✿ ⅓ cup coconut cream
- ✿ 3 tablespoons Kalamata olives, pitted
- ✿ 2 teaspoons melted butter
- ✿ ⅓ teaspoon ground black pepper
- ✿ 2 cloves garlic, peeled
- ✿ Pinch of freshly grated nutmeg
- ✿ Sea salt, to taste
- ✿ 2 tablespoons smoked paprika powder

1. Pour the water into the Instant Pot and put the steamer basket in the pot. Place the cauliflower florets in the steamer basket.
2. Close and secure the lid. Select the Manual mode and set the cooking time for 2 minutes at High Pressure. Once cooking is complete, do a quick pressure release. Carefully open the lid.
3. In a blender, combine the cooked cauliflower along with the remaining ingredients, except for the smoked paprika powder. Pulse until puréed.
4. Form the cauliflower mixture into balls and roll each ball into the smoked paprika powder. Arrange on the serving platters. Serve immediately.

Per Serving
calories: 67 | fat: 5.2g | protein: 1.8g | carbs: 5.0g | net carbs: 2.9g | fiber: 2.1g

Cabbage in Cream Sauce

Prep time: 10 minutes | Cook time: 13 minutes | Serves 4

- 1 tablespoon unsalted butter
- ½ cup diced pancetta
- ¼ cup diced yellow onion
- 1 cup chicken broth
- 1 pound (454 g) green cabbage, finely chopped
- 1 bay leaf
- ⅓ cup heavy cream
- 1 tablespoon dried parsley
- 1 teaspoon fine grind sea salt
- ¼ teaspoon ground nutmeg
- ¼ teaspoon ground black pepper

1. Press the Sauté button on the Instant Pot and melt the butter. Add the pancetta and onion to the pot and sauté for about 4 minutes, or until the onion is tender and begins to brown.
2. Pour in the chicken broth. Using a wooden spoon, stir and loosen any browned bits from the bottom of the pot. Stir in the cabbage and bay leaf.
3. Lock the lid. Select the Manual mode and set the cooking time for 4 minutes on High Pressure. When the timer goes off, perform a quick pressure release. Carefully open the lid.
4. Select Sauté mode and bring the ingredients to a boil. Stir in the remaining ingredients and simmer for 5 additional minutes.
5. Remove and discard the bay leaf. Spoon into serving bowls. Serve warm.

Per Serving

calories: 211 | fat: 17.1g | protein: 7.2g | carbs: 7.3g | net carbs: 5.0g | fiber: 2.3g

Garlicky Buttery Whole Cauliflower

Prep time: 5 minutes | Cook time: 8 minutes | Serves 4

- 1 large cauliflower, rinsed and patted dry
- 1 cup water
- 4 tablespoons melted butter
- 2 cloves garlic, minced
- Pinch of sea salt
- Pinch of fresh ground black pepper
- 1 tablespoon chopped fresh flat leaf parsley, for garnish

1. Pour the water into the Instant Pot and put the trivet in the pot. Place the cauliflower on the trivet.
2. Lock the lid. Select the Manual mode and set the cooking time for 3 minutes at High Pressure.
3. Preheat the oven to 550ºF (288ºC). Line a baking sheet with parchment paper.
4. In a small bowl, whisk together the butter, garlic, sea salt and black pepper. Set aside.
5. When the timer beeps, use a quick pressure release. Carefully open the lid.
6. Transfer the cauliflower to the lined baking sheet. Dab and dry the surface with a clean kitchen towel. Brush the cauliflower with the garlic butter.
7. Place the baking sheet with the cauliflower in the preheated oven and roast for 5 minutes, or until the cauliflower is golden brown. Drizzle with any remaining garlic butter and sprinkle with the chopped parsley. Serve immediately.

Per Serving

calories: 141 | fat: 12.3g | protein: 3.1g | carbs: 7.9g | net carbs: 4.2g | fiber: 3.7g

Stir-Fried Cauliflower Rice with Mushrooms

Prep time: 10 minutes | Cook time: 13 minutes | Serves 4

- ✿ 1 medium head cauliflower, cut into florets
- ✿ 1 cup water
- ✿ 1½ tablespoons unsalted butter
- ✿ 3 garlic cloves, minced
- ✿ 1 cup sliced fresh white mushrooms
- ✿ 1 teaspoon coconut aminos
- ✿ 1½ tablespoons olive oil
- ✿ 1 large egg, beaten
- ✿ ¼ teaspoon fine grind sea salt
- ✿ ⅛ teaspoon ground black pepper
- ✿ ½ tablespoon chopped fresh flat-leaf parsley

1. Place a steamer basket with legs in the inner pot and pour the water in the pot. Place the cauliflower florets in the steamer basket.
2. Lock the lid. Select the Steam mode and set the cooking time for 3 minutes on High Pressure. When the timer goes off, perform a quick pressure release. Carefully open the lid.
3. Transfer the cauliflower florets to a blender. Pulse until it reaches a rice-like texture. Set aside.
4. Remove the steamer basket from the pot. Pour out the water and wipe the pot dry with a paper towel.
5. Select Sauté setting and melt the butter. Add the garlic and mushrooms to the pot and sauté for 4 minutes, or until the mushrooms are tender.
6. Stir in the coconut aminos, olive oil and cauliflower rice. Sauté for 3 minutes.
7. Whisk in the beaten egg and sauté for 3 minutes, or until the egg is thoroughly cooked. Season with the sea salt and black pepper and stir to combine.
8. Transfer the fried rice to serving bowls and sprinkle the parsley on top. Serve hot.

Per Serving
calories: 131 | fat: 9.1g | protein: 5.2g | carbs: 7.1g | net carbs: 5.0g | fiber: 2.1g

Spinach with Almonds and Olives

Prep time: 15 minutes | Cook time: 2 to 3 minutes | Serves 4

- ✿ 1 tablespoon olive oil
- ✿ 3 cloves garlic, smashed
- ✿ Bunch scallions, chopped
- ✿ 2 pounds (907 g) spinach, washed
- ✿ 1 cup vegetable broth
- ✿ 1 tablespoon champagne vinegar
- ✿ ½ teaspoon dried dill weed
- ✿ ¼ teaspoon cayenne pepper
- ✿ Seasoned salt and ground black pepper, to taste
- ✿ ½ cup almonds, soaked overnight and drained
- ✿ 2 tablespoons green olives, pitted and halved
- ✿ 2 tablespoons water
- ✿ 1 tablespoon extra-virgin olive oil
- ✿ 2 teaspoons lemon juice
- ✿ 1 teaspoon garlic powder
- ✿ 1 teaspoon onion powder

1. Press the Sauté button on the Instant Pot and heat the olive oil. Add the garlic and scallions to the pot and sauté for 1 to 2 minutes, or until fragrant.
2. Stir in the spinach, vegetable broth, vinegar, dill, cayenne pepper, salt and black pepper.
3. Lock the lid. Select the Manual mode and set the cooking time for 1 minute on High Pressure. When the timer goes off, perform a quick pressure release. Carefully open the lid.
4. Stir in the remaining ingredients.
5. Transfer to serving plates and serve immediately.

Per Serving
calories: 239 | fat: 16.9g | protein: 11.1g | carbs: 17.0g | net carbs: 8.7g | fiber: 8.3g

Zoodles with Mediterranean Sauce

Prep time: 10 minutes | Cook time: 5 minutes | Serves 2

- ✿ 1 tablespoon olive oil
- ✿ 2 tomatoes, chopped
- ✿ ½ cup water
- ✿ ½ cup roughly chopped fresh parsley
- ✿ 3 tablespoons ground almonds
- ✿ 1 tablespoon fresh rosemary, chopped
- ✿ 1 tablespoon apple cider vinegar
- ✿ 1 teaspoon garlic, smashed
- ✿ 2 zucchinis, spiralized and cooked
- ✿ ½ avocado, pitted and sliced
- ✿ Salt and ground black pepper, to taste

1. Add the olive oil, tomatoes, water, parsley, ground almonds, rosemary, apple cider vinegar and garlic to the Instant Pot.
2. Lock the lid. Select the Manual mode and set the cooking time for 5 minutes on High Pressure. When the timer beeps, perform a natural pressure release for 10 minutes, then release any remaining pressure. Carefully open the lid.
3. Divide the cooked zucchini spirals between two serving plates. Spoon the sauce over each serving. Top with the avocado slices and season with salt and black pepper.
4. Serve immediately.

Per Serving

calories: 264 | fat: 20.0g | protein: 7.2g | carbs: 19.6g | net carbs: 10.7g | fiber: 8.9g

Peppery Brussels Sprouts

Prep time: 10 minutes | Cook time: 7 minutes | Serves 4

- ✿ 2 tablespoons olive oil
- ✿ 1 white onion, chopped
- ✿ ¾ pound (340 g) Brussels sprouts, trimmed and halved
- ✿ 1 red bell pepper, deseeded and chopped
- ✿ 1 habanero pepper, chopped
- ✿ 1 cup vegetable broth
- ✿ 1 cup water
- ✿ 2 tablespoons unsweetened tomato purée
- ✿ 1 tablespoon coconut aminos
- ✿ 1 teaspoon fennel seeds
- ✿ ½ teaspoon paprika
- ✿ 2 bay leaves
- ✿ 1 garlic clove, minced
- ✿ Sea salt and freshly ground black pepper, to taste

1. Press the Sauté button on the Instant Pot and heat the oil. Add the onion to the pot and sauté for 3 minutes, or until tender. Stir in the remaining ingredients.
2. Lock the lid. Select the Manual mode and set the cooking time for 4 minutes on Low Pressure. When the timer goes off, perform a quick pressure release. Carefully open the lid.
3. Remove and discard the bay leaves. Serve warm.

Per Serving

calories: 130 | fat: 7.3g | protein: 4.5g | carbs: 15.1g | net carbs: 10.4g | fiber: 4.7g

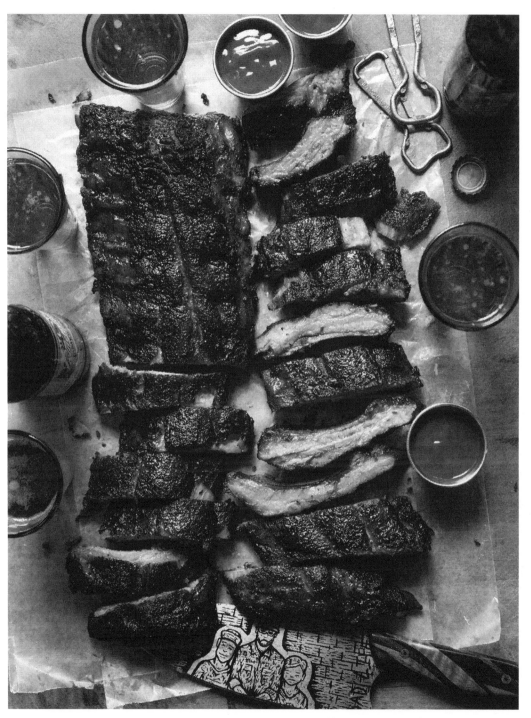

CHAPTER 6
Beef and Lamb

Beef Back Ribs with Barbecue Glaze

Prep time: 10 minutes | Cook time: 35 minutes | Serves 4

- ½ cup water
- 1 (3-pound / 1.4-kg) rack beef back ribs, prepared with rub of choice
- ¼ cup unsweetened tomato purée
- ¼ teaspoon Worcestershire sauce
- ¼ teaspoon garlic powder
- 2 teaspoons apple cider vinegar
- ¼ teaspoon liquid smoke
- ¼ teaspoon smoked paprika
- 3 tablespoons Swerve
- Dash of cayenne pepper

1. Pour the water in the pot and place the trivet inside.
2. Arrange the ribs on top of the trivet.
3. Close the lid. Select Manual mode and set cooking time for 25 minutes on High Pressure.
4. Meanwhile, prepare the glaze by whisking together the tomato purée, Worcestershire sauce, garlic powder, vinegar, liquid smoke, paprika, Swerve, and cayenne in a medium bowl. Heat the broiler.
5. When timer beeps, quick release the pressure. Open the lid. Remove the ribs and place on a baking sheet.
6. Brush a layer of glaze on the ribs. Put under the broiler for 5 minutes.
7. Remove from the broiler and brush with glaze again. Put back under the broiler for 5 more minutes, or until the tops are sticky.
8. Serve immediately.

Per Serving
calories: 758 | fat: 26.8g | protein: 33.7g | carbs: 0.9g | net carbs: 0.7g | fiber: 0.2g

Harissa Lamb

Prep time: 30 minutes | Cook time: 40 minutes | Serves 4

- 1 tablespoon keto-friendly Harissa sauce
- 1 teaspoon dried thyme
- ½ teaspoon salt
- 1 pound (454 g) lamb shoulder
- 2 tablespoons sesame oil
- 2 cups water

1. In a bowl, mix the Harissa, dried thyme, and salt.
2. Rub the lamb shoulder with the Harissa mixture and brush with sesame oil.
3. Heat the the Instant Pot on Sauté mode for 2 minutes and put the lamb shoulder inside.
4. Cook the lamb for 3 minutes on each side, then pour in the water.
5. Close the lid. Select Manual mode and set cooking time for 40 minutes on High Pressure.
6. When timer beeps, use a natural pressure release for 25 minutes, then release any remaining pressure. Open the lid.
7. Serve warm.

Per Serving
calories: 284 | fat: 15.8g | protein: 32.1g | carbs: 1.7g | net carbs: 1.6g | fiber: 0.1g

Beef Brisket with Cabbage

Prep time: 15 minutes | Cook time: 1 hour 7 minutes | Serves 8

- ✿ 3 pounds (1.4 kg) corned beef brisket
- ✿ 4 cups water
- ✿ 3 garlic cloves, minced
- ✿ 2 teaspoons yellow mustard seed
- ✿ 2 teaspoons black peppercorns
- ✿ 3 celery stalks, chopped
- ✿ ½ large white onion, chopped
- ✿ 1 green cabbage, cut into quarters

1. Add the brisket to the Instant Pot. Pour the water into the pot. Add the garlic, mustard seed, and black peppercorns.
2. Lock the lid. Select Meat/Stew mode and set cooking time for 50 minutes on High Pressure.
3. When cooking is complete, allow the pressure to release naturally for 20 minutes, then release any remaining pressure. Open the lid and transfer only the brisket to a platter.
4. Add the celery, onion, and cabbage to the pot.
5. Lock the lid. Select Soup mode and set cooking time for 12 minutes on High Pressure.
6. When cooking is complete, quick release the pressure. Open the lid, add the brisket back to the pot and let warm in the pot for 5 minutes.
7. Transfer the warmed brisket back to the platter and thinly slice. Transfer the vegetables to the platter. Serve hot.

Per Serving

calories: 357 | fat: 25.5g | protein: 26.3g | carbs: 7.3g | net carbs: 5.3g | fiber: 2.0g

Beef Carne Guisada

Prep time: 10 minutes | Cook time: 20 minutes | Serves 4

- ✿ 2 tomatoes, chopped
- ✿ 1 red bell pepper, chopped
- ✿ ½ onion, chopped
- ✿ 3 garlic cloves, chopped
- ✿ 1 teaspoon ancho chili powder
- ✿ 1 tablespoon ground cumin
- ✿ ½ teaspoon dried oregano
- ✿ 1 teaspoons salt
- ✿ 1 teaspoon freshly ground black pepper
- ✿ 1 teaspoon smoked paprika
- ✿ 1 pound (454 g) beef chuck, cut into large pieces
- ✿ ¾ cup water, plus 2 tablespoons
- ✿ ¼ teaspoon xanthan gum

1. In a blender, purée the tomatoes, bell pepper, onion, garlic, chili powder, cumin, oregano, salt, pepper, and paprika.
2. Put the beef pieces in the Instant Pot. Pour in the blended mixture.
3. Use ¾ cup of water to wash out the blender and pour the liquid into the pot.
4. Lock the lid. Select Manual mode and set cooking time for 20 minutes on High Pressure.
5. When cooking is complete, quick release the pressure. Unlock the lid.
6. Switch the pot to Sauté mode. Bring the stew to a boil.
7. Put the xanthan gum and 2 tablespoons of water into the boiling stew and stir until it thickens.
8. Serve immediately.

Per Serving

calories: 326 | fat: 22.0g | protein: 23.0g | carbs: 9.0g | net carbs: 7.0g | fiber: 2.0g

Beef Masala Curry

Prep time: 10 minutes | Cook time: 20 minutes | Serves 4

- ✿ 2 tomatoes, quartered
- ✿ 1 small onion, quartered
- ✿ 4 garlic cloves, chopped
- ✿ ½ cup fresh cilantro leaves
- ✿ 1 teaspoon garam masala
- ✿ ½ teaspoon ground coriander
- ✿ 1 teaspoon ground cumin
- ✿ ½ teaspoon cayenne
- ✿ 1 teaspoon salt
- ✿ 1 pound (454 g) beef chuck roast, cut into 1-inch cubes

1. In a blender, combine the tomatoes, onion, garlic, and cilantro.
2. Process until the vegetables are puréed. Add the garam masala, coriander, cumin, cayenne, and salt. Process for several more seconds.
3. To the Instant Pot, add the beef and pour the vegetable purée on top.
4. Lock the lid. Select Manual mode and set cooking time for 20 minutes on High Pressure.
5. When timer beeps, let the pressure release naturally for 10 minutes, then release any remaining pressure. Unlock the lid.
6. Stir and serve immediately.

Per Serving

calories: 309 | fat: 21.0g | protein: 24.0g | carbs: 6.0g | net carbs: 4.0g | fiber: 2.0g

Beef Shawarma and Veggie Salad Bowls

Prep time: 10 minutes | Cook time: 19 minutes | Serves 4

- ✿ 2 teaspoons olive oil
- ✿ 1½ pounds (680 g) beef flank steak, thinly sliced
- ✿ Sea salt and freshly ground black pepper, to taste
- ✿ 1 teaspoon cayenne pepper
- ✿ ½ teaspoon ground bay leaf
- ✿ ½ teaspoon ground allspice
- ✿ ½ teaspoon cumin, divided
- ✿ ½ cup Greek yogurt
- ✿ 2 tablespoons sesame oil
- ✿ 1 tablespoon fresh lime juice
- ✿ 2 English cucumbers, chopped
- ✿ 1 cup cherry tomatoes, halved
- ✿ 1 red onion, thinly sliced
- ✿ ½ head romaine lettuce, chopped

1. Press the Sauté button to heat up the Instant Pot. Then, heat the olive oil and cook the beef for about 4 minutes.
2. Add all seasonings, 1½ cups of water, and secure the lid.
3. Choose Manual mode. Set the cook time for 15 minutes on High Pressure.
4. Once cooking is complete, use a natural pressure release. Carefully remove the lid.
5. Allow the beef to cool completely.
6. To make the dressing, whisk Greek yogurt, sesame oil, and lime juice in a mixing bowl.
7. Then, divide cucumbers, tomatoes, red onion, and romaine lettuce among four serving bowls. Dress the salad and top with the reserved beef flank steak. Serve warm.

Per Serving

calories: 367 | fat: 19.1g | protein: 39.5g | carbs: 8.4g | net carbs: 5.0g | fiber: 3.4g

Lamb Kofta Curry

Prep time: 15 minutes | Cook time: 20 minutes | Serves 4

- ✿ 1 pound (454 g) ground lamb
- ✿ 4 ounces (113 g) scallions, chopped
- ✿ 1 tablespoon curry powder, divided
- ✿ ½ teaspoon chili flakes
- ✿ 1 tablespoon dried cilantro
- ✿ 1 tablespoon coconut oil
- ✿ 1 cup chicken broth
- ✿ ⅓ cup coconut cream

1. In a mixing bowl, mix the ground lamb, scallions, and ½ tablespoon of curry powder.
2. Add chili flakes and dried cilantro. Stir the mixture until homogenous and shape the mixture into medium size koftas (meatballs).
3. Heat the coconut oil in the Instant Pot on Sauté mode until melted.
4. Put the koftas in the hot oil and cook for 2 minutes on each side.
5. Meanwhile, mix the chicken broth, coconut cream and remaining curry powder in a small bowl.
6. Pour the mixture over the koftas.
7. Select Manual mode and set timer for 12 minutes on High Pressure.
8. When timer beeps, use a natural pressure release for 10 minutes, then release any remaining pressure. Open the lid.
9. Serve warm.

Per Serving

calories: 310 | fat: 17.1g | protein: 34.2g | carbs: 4.4g | net carbs: 2.7g | fiber: 1.7g

Galbijjim

Prep time: 10 minutes | Cook time: 12 minutes | Serves 8

- ✿ 2 pounds (907 g) meaty short ribs
- ✿ 2 tablespoons gochujang
- ✿ 4 garlic cloves, crushed
- ✿ 1 tablespoon mirin
- ✿ 3 tablespoons coconut aminos
- ✿ 2 teaspoons minced fresh ginger
- ✿ 1 teaspoon Swerve
- ✿ ¼ teaspoon powdered stevia
- ✿ 1 teaspoon salt
- ✿ 2 teaspoons freshly ground black pepper
- ✿ 1 tablespoon sesame oil
- ✿ ¼ cup water
- ✿ ¼ teaspoon xanthan gum

1. Put the ribs into a large zip-top bag. Whisk in the remaining ingredients, except for the water and xanthan gum.
2. Shake to coat the ribs well and seal the bag. Marinate the ribs in the refrigerator for at least 1 hour.
3. Put the ribs and marinade in the Instant Pot along with the water.
4. Lock the lid. Select Manual mode and set cooking time for 12 minutes on High Pressure.
5. When cooking is complete, let the pressure release naturally for 5 minutes, then release any remaining pressure. Unlock the lid.
6. Turn the Instant Pot on Sauté mode. Transfer the ribs to a platter. Bring the sauce to a boil, then fold in the xanthan gum and stir until the sauce thickens.
7. Pour the sauce over the ribs and serve.

Per Serving

calories: 467 | fat: 43.0g | protein: 17.0g | carbs: 3.0g | net carbs: 3.0g | fiber: 0g

Lamb Rostelle

Prep time: 20 minutes | Cook time: 30 minutes | Serves 4

- ✿ 1 pound (454 g) lamb loin, slice into strips
- ✿ ½ teaspoon apple cider vinegar
- ✿ 1 teaspoon ground black pepper
- ✿ 1 teaspoon olive oil
- ✿ ½ teaspoon salt
- ✿ 1 cup water, for cooking

1. Combine the apple cider vinegar, ground black pepper, olive oil, and salt in a bowl. Stir to mix well.
2. Put the lamb strips in the bowl and toss to coat well.
3. Run the lamb strips through four skewers and put in a baking pan.
4. Pour water in the Instant Pot and then insert the trivet.
5. Put the baking pan on the trivet. Close the lid.
6. Select Manual mode and set cooking time for 30 minutes on High Pressure.
7. When timer beeps, use a natural pressure release for 10 minutes, then release any remaining pressure. Open the lid.
8. Serve immediately.

Per Serving
calories: 241 | fat: 12.3g | protein: 30.2g | carbs: 0.4g | net carbs: 0.3g | fiber: 0.1g

---

Beef Ribs with Radishes

Prep time: 20 minutes | Cook time: 56 minutes | Serves 4

- ✿ ¼ teaspoon ground coriander
- ✿ ¼ teaspoon ground cumin
- ✿ 1 teaspoon kosher salt, plus more to taste
- ✿ ½ teaspoon smoked paprika
- ✿ Pinch of ground allspice (optional)
- ✿ 4 (8-ounce / 227-g) bone-in beef short ribs
- ✿ 2 tablespoons avocado oil
- ✿ 1 cup water
- ✿ 2 radishes, ends trimmed, leaves rinsed and roughly chopped
- ✿ Freshly ground black pepper, to taste

1. In a small bowl, mix together the coriander, cumin, salt, paprika, and allspice. Rub the spice mixture all over the short ribs.
2. Set the Instant Pot to Sauté mode and add the oil to heat. Add the short ribs, bone side up. Brown for 4 minutes on each side.
3. Pour the water into the Instant Pot. Secure the lid. Press the Manual button and set cooking time for 45 minutes on High Pressure.
4. When timer beeps, allow the pressure to release naturally for 10 minutes, then release any remaining pressure. Open the lid.
5. Remove the short ribs to a serving plate.
6. Add the radishes to the sauce in the pot. Place a metal steaming basket directly on top of the radishes and place the radish leaves in the basket.
7. Secure the lid. Press the Manual button and set cooking time for 3 minutes on High Pressure.
8. When timer beeps, quick release the pressure. Open the lid. Transfer the leaves to a serving bowl. Sprinkle with with salt and pepper.
9. Remove the radishes and place on top of the leaves. Serve hot with the short ribs.

Per Serving
calories: 450 | fat: 24.8g | protein: 45.4g | carbs: 12.3g | net carbs: 9.4g | fiber: 2.9g

Classic Osso Buco with Gremolata

Prep time: 35 minutes | Cook time: 1 hour 2 minutes | Serves 6

- 4 bone-in beef shanks
- Sea salt, to taste
- 2 tablespoons avocado oil
- 1 small turnip, diced
- 1 medium onion, diced
- 1 medium stalk celery, diced
- 4 cloves garlic, smashed
- 1 tablespoon unsweetened tomato purée
- ½ cup dry white wine
- 1 cup chicken broth
- 1 sprig fresh rosemary
- 2 sprigs fresh thyme
- 3 Roma tomatoes, diced

For the Gremolata:
- ½ cup loosely packed parsley leaves
- 1 clove garlic, crushed
- Grated zest of 2 lemons

1. On a clean work surface, season the shanks all over with salt.
2. Set the Instant Pot to Sauté and add the oil. When the oil shimmers, add 2 shanks and sear for 4 minutes per side. Remove the shanks to a bowl and repeat with the remaining shanks. Set aside.
3. Add the turnip, onion, and celery to the pot and cook for 5 minutes or until softened.
4. Add the garlic and unsweetened tomato purée and cook 1 minute more, stirring frequently.
5. Deglaze the pot with the wine, scraping the bottom with a wooden spoon to loosen any browned bits. Bring to a boil.
6. Add the broth, rosemary, thyme, and shanks, then add the tomatoes on top of the shanks.
7. Secure the lid. Press the Manual button and set cooking time for 40 minutes on High Pressure.
8. Meanwhile, for the gremolata: In a small food processor, combine the parsley, garlic, and lemon zest and pulse until the parsley is finely chopped. Refrigerate until ready to use.
9. When timer beeps, allow the pressure to release naturally for 20 minutes, then release any remaining pressure. Open the lid.
10. To serve, transfer the shanks to large, shallow serving bowl. Ladle the braising sauce over the top and sprinkle with the gremolata.

Per Serving
calories: 605 | fat: 30.1g | protein: 69.1g | carbs: 7.7g | net carbs: 6.0g | fiber: 1.7g

Beef Shoulder Roast

Prep time: 15 minutes | Cook time: 46 minutes | Serves 6

- 2 tablespoons peanut oil
- 2 pounds (907 g) shoulder roast
- ¼ cup coconut aminos
- 1 teaspoon porcini powder
- 1 teaspoon garlic powder
- 1 cup beef broth
- 2 cloves garlic, minced
- 2 tablespoons champagne vinegar
- ½ teaspoon hot sauce
- 1 teaspoon celery seeds
- 1 cup purple onions, cut into wedges
- 1 tablespoon flaxseed meal, plus 2 tablespoons water

1. Press the Sauté button to heat up the Instant Pot. Then, heat the peanut oil and cook the beef shoulder roast for 3 minutes on each side.
2. In a mixing dish, combine coconut aminos, porcini powder, garlic powder, broth, garlic, vinegar, hot sauce, and celery seeds.
3. Pour the broth mixture into the Instant Pot. Add the onions to the top.
4. Secure the lid. Choose Meat/Stew mode and set cooking time for 40 minutes on High Pressure.
5. Once cooking is complete, use a natural pressure release for 15 minutes, then release any remaining pressure. Carefully remove the lid.
6. Make the slurry by mixing flaxseed meal with 2 tablespoons of water. Add the slurry to the Instant Pot.
7. Press the Sauté button and allow it to cook until the cooking liquid is reduced and thickened slightly. Serve warm.

Per Serving
calories: 313 | fat: 16.1g | protein: 33.5g | carbs: 6.5g | net carbs: 3.1g | fiber: 3.4g

Beef, Bacon and Cauliflower Rice Casserole

Prep time: 15 minutes | Cook time: 26 minutes | Serves 5

- ✿ 2 cups fresh cauliflower florets
- ✿ 1 pound (454 g) ground beef
- ✿ 5 slices uncooked bacon, chopped
- ✿ 8 ounces (227 g) unsweetened tomato purée
- ✿ 1 cup shredded Cheddar cheese, divided
- ✿ 1 teaspoon garlic powder
- ✿ ½ teaspoon paprika
- ✿ ½ teaspoon sea salt
- ✿ ¼ teaspoon ground black pepper
- ✿ ¼ teaspoon celery seed
- ✿ 1 cup water
- ✿ 1 medium Roma tomato, sliced

1. Spray a round soufflé dish with coconut oil cooking spray. Set aside.
2. Add the cauliflower florets to a food processor and pulse until a riced. Set aside.
3. Select Sauté mode. Once the pot is hot, crumble the ground beef into the pot and add the bacon. Sauté for 6 minutes or until the ground beef is browned and the bacon is cooked through.
4. Transfer the beef, bacon, and rendered fat to a large bowl.
5. Add the cauliflower rice, tomato purée, ½ cup Cheddar cheese, garlic powder, paprika, sea salt, black pepper, and celery seed to the bowl with the beef and bacon. Mix well to combine.
6. Add the mixture to the prepared dish and use a spoon to press and smooth the mixture into an even layer.
7. Place the trivet in the Instant Pot and add the water to the bottom of the pot. Place the dish on top of the trivet.
8. Lock the lid. Select Manual mode and set cooking time for 20 minutes on High Pressure.
9. When cooking is complete, quick release the pressure.
10. Open the lid. Arrange the tomato slices in a single layer on top of the casserole and sprinkle the remaining cheese over top.
11. Secure the lid and let the residual heat melt the cheese for 5 minutes.
12. Open the lid, remove the dish from the pot.
13. Transfer the casserole to a serving plate and slice into 5 equal-sized wedges. Serve warm.

Per Serving
calories: 350 | fat: 22.7g | protein: 30.0g | carbs: 8.0g | net carbs: 6.0g | fiber: 2.0g

Braised Tri-Tip Steak

Prep time: 20 minutes | Cook time: 54 minutes | Serves 4

- ✿ 2 pounds (907 g) tri-tip steak, patted dry
- ✿ 2 teaspoons coarse sea salt
- ✿ 3 tablespoons avocado oil
- ✿ ½ medium onion, diced
- ✿ 2 cloves garlic, smashed
- ✿ 1 tablespoon unsweetened tomato purée
- ✿ 1½ cups dry red wine
- ✿ ½ tablespoon dried thyme
- ✿ 2 bay leaves
- ✿ 1 Roma (plum) tomato, diced
- ✿ 1 stalk celery, including leaves, chopped
- ✿ 1 small turnip, chopped
- ✿ ½ cup water

1. Season the tri-tip with the coarse salt. Set the Instant Pot to Sauté mode and heat the avocado oil until shimmering.
2. Cook the steak in the pot for 2 minutes per side or until well browned. Remove the steak from the pot and place it in a shallow bowl. Set aside.
3. Add the onion to the pot and sauté for 3 minutes. Add the garlic and sauté for 1 minute. Add the unsweetened tomato purée and cook for 1 minute, stirring constantly.
4. Pour in the red wine. Stir in the thyme and bay leaves.
5. Return the tri-tip steak to the pot. Scatter the tomato, celery, and turnip around the steak. Pour in the water.
6. Secure the lid. Press the Manual button and set cooking time for 35 minutes on High Pressure.
7. When timer beeps, allow the pressure to release naturally for 20 minutes, then release any remaining pressure. Open the lid. Discard the bay leaves.
8. Remove the steak and place in a dish. Press the Sauté button and bring the braising liquid to a boil. Cook for 10 minutes or until the liquid is reduced by about half.
9. Slice the steak thinly and serve with braising liquid over.

Per Serving
calories: 726 | fat: 45.1g | protein: 68.7g | carbs: 3.5g | net carbs: 2.6g | fiber: 0.9g

Cheesy Bacon Stuffed Meatloaf

Prep time: 15 minutes | Cook time: 32 minutes | Serves 4

- 1 pound (454 g) ground beef
- 1 large egg, beaten
- ½ cup unsweetened tomato purée
- 2 tablespoons golden flaxseed meal
- 1 teaspoon garlic powder
- 1 teaspoon sea salt

- ½ teaspoon paprika
- ¼ teaspoon ground black pepper
- 4 slices uncooked bacon
- ⅓ cup shredded Cheddar cheese
- 1 cup water

For The Glaze:

- ⅓ cup unsweetened tomato purée
- 1 teaspoon apple cider vinegar
- ¼ teaspoon onion powder
- ¼ teaspoon garlic powder

- 2 teaspoons erythritol
- ⅛ teaspoon sea salt
- ⅛ teaspoon allspice

1. In a large bowl, combine the ground beef, egg, tomato purée, flaxseed meal, garlic powder, sea salt, paprika, and black pepper. Mix to combine well.
2. Place a sheet of aluminum foil on a flat surface. Place half of the meat mixture in the center of the foil sheet and use the hands to mold the mixture into a flat oval shape that is about 6 inches long.
3. Place the bacon slices on top of the meat and sprinkle the Cheddar over. Place the remaining meat mixture on top and shape the mixture into an oval-shaped loaf.
4. Fold the sides of the foil up and around the sides of the meatloaf to form a loaf pan. Set aside.
5. Make the tomato glaze by combining the tomato purée, vinegar, onion powder, garlic powder, erythritol, sea salt, and allspice in a small bowl. Mix well. Spoon the glaze over the meatloaf.
6. Add the water to the Instant Pot. Place the loaf on the trivet and lower the trivet into the pot.
7. Lock the lid. Select Manual mode and set cooking time for 30 minutes on High Pressure.
8. While the meatloaf is cooking, preheat the oven broiler to 550°F (288°C).
9. When cooking time is complete, quick release the pressure, then open the lid and carefully remove the meatloaf from the pot.
10. Transfer the loaf pan to a large baking sheet. Place the meatloaf under the broiler to brown for 2 minutes or until the glaze is bubbling.
11. Transfer the browned meatloaf to a serving plate, discard the foil, and cut the loaf into 8 equal-sized slices. Serve hot.

Per Serving

calories: 395 | fat: 27.3g | protein: 40.0g | carbs: 5.5g | net carbs: 3.4g | fiber: 2.1g

Classic and Sumptuous Pot Roast

Prep time: 15 minutes | Cook time: 1 hour 8 minutes | Serves 6

- ¼ cup dry red wine
- 1 tablespoon dried thyme
- 1½ cups beef broth
- ½ tablespoon dried rosemary
- 1 teaspoon paprika
- 1 teaspoon garlic powder
- 1½ teaspoons sea salt
- ½ teaspoon ground black pepper
- 3 pounds (1.4 kg) boneless chuck roast

- 1½ tablespoons avocado oil
- 2 tablespoons unsalted butter
- ½ medium yellow onion, chopped
- 2 garlic cloves, minced
- 1 cup sliced mushrooms
- 4 stalks celery, chopped
- 2 sprigs fresh thyme
- 1 bay leaf

1. In a medium bowl, combine the wine, dried thyme, beef broth, and dried rosemary. Stir to combine. Set aside.
2. In a small bowl, combine the paprika, garlic powder, sea salt, and black pepper. Mix well. Generously rub the dry spice mixture into the roast. Set aside.
3. Select Sauté mode. Once the pot becomes hot, add the avocado oil and butter and heat until the butter is melted, about 2 minutes.
4. Add the roast to the pot. Sauté for 3 minutes per side or until a crust is formed. Transfer the browned roast to a plate and set aside.
5. Add the onions and garlic to the pot. Sauté for 3 minutes or until the onions soften and the garlic becomes fragrant.
6. Add half the broth and wine mixture to the pot.
7. Place the trivet in the Instant Pot and place the roast on top of the trivet. Add the mushrooms and celery to the pot, and pour the remaining broth and wine mixture over the roast. Place the thyme sprigs and bay leaf on top of the roast.
8. Lock the lid. Select Manual mode and set cooking time for 1 hour on High Pressure.
9. When cooking is complete, allow the pressure to release naturally for 10 minutes and then release the remaining pressure.
10. Open the lid, discard the bay leaf and thyme sprigs. Transfer the roast to a serving platter.
11. Transfer the vegetables to the platter and spoon the remaining broth over the roast and vegetables.
12. Slice the roast and ladle ¼ cup of the broth over each serving. Serve hot.

Per Serving

calories: 403 | fat: 21.2g | protein: 49.8g | carbs: 4.1g | net carbs: 3.1g | fiber: 1.0g

Hearty Chimichurri Skirt Steak

Prep time: 15 minutes | Cook time: 30 minutes | Serves 4

- 1 pound (454 g) skirt steak, trimmed and cut into 4 equal-sized pieces
- ½ teaspoon sea salt
- ½ teaspoon black pepper
- 1 tablespoon avocado oil
- 1 cup water

Chimichurri:

- ⅓ cup chopped flat-leaf parsley
- 3 large garlic cloves, minced
- 2½ tablespoons red wine vinegar
- ½ teaspoon dried oregano
- ¼ teaspoon crushed red pepper
- ½ teaspoon sea salt
- ½ teaspoon black pepper
- 1 teaspoon lemon juice
- ½ cup extra virgin olive oil

1. Add the parsley to a food processor and pulse until finely chopped. Add the garlic, red wine vinegar, oregano, crushed red pepper, ½ teaspoon sea salt, ½ teaspoon black pepper, and lemon juice. Pulse until combined. Add the olive oil and pulse until the ingredients are well blended. Set aside.
2. Season both sides of the steaks with the remaining salt and pepper.
3. Select Sauté mode. Once the Instant Pot is hot, add the avocado oil and let heat for 1 minute.
4. Add the steaks to the pot, two at a time, and sauté for 2 minutes per side or until browned on both sides. Transfer the browned steaks to a plate and repeat with the remaining steaks.
5. Place one sheet on a flat surface. Place two steaks in the center of the sheet and pour half the chimichurri sauce over top of the steaks. Place the remaining steaks on top and pour the remaining sauce over top.
6. Place another sheet of foil over the steaks and tightly roll and crimp the ends to create a foil packet.
7. Place the trivet in the pot and add the water to the bottom of the pot. Place the foil packet on top of the trivet.
8. Lock the lid. Select Manual mode and set cooking time for 25 minutes on High Pressure.
9. When cooking is complete, allow the pressure to release naturally for 6 minutes and then release the remaining pressure.
10. Open the lid, remove the steaks from the pot. Set the steaks aside to rest for 2 minutes.
11. Open the packet and transfer the steaks to a cutting board. Thinly slice and transfer to a serving platter. Serve warm.

Per Serving
calories: 508 | fat: 42.1g | protein: 31.9g | carbs: 1.7g | net carbs: 1.3g | fiber: 0.4g

Beef Cheeseburger Pie

Prep time: 15 minutes | Cook time: 30 minutes | Serves 6

- 1 tablespoon olive oil
- 1 pound (454 g) ground beef
- 3 eggs (1 beaten)
- ½ cup unsweetened tomato purée
- 2 tablespoons golden flaxseed meal
- 1 garlic clove, minced
- ½ teaspoon Italian seasoning blend
- ½ teaspoon sea salt
- ½ teaspoon smoked paprika
- ½ teaspoon onion powder
- 2 tablespoons heavy cream
- ½ teaspoon ground mustard
- ¼ teaspoon ground black pepper
- 2 cups water
- ½ cup grated Cheddar cheese

1. Coat a round cake pan with the olive oil.
2. Select Sauté mode. Once the pot is hot, add the ground beef and sauté for 5 minutes or until the beef is browned.
3. Transfer the beef to a large bowl.
4. Add the 1 beaten egg, tomato purée, flaxseed meal, garlic, Italian seasoning, sea salt, smoked paprika, and onion powder to the bowl. Mix until well combined.
5. Transfer the meat mixture to the prepared cake pan and use a knife to spread the mixture into an even layer. Set aside.
6. In a separate medium bowl, combine the 2 remaining eggs, heavy cream, ground mustard, and black pepper. Whisk until combined.
7. Pour the egg mixture over the meat mixture. Tightly cover the pan with a sheet of aluminum foil.
8. Place the trivet in the Instant Pot and add the water to the bottom of the pot. Place the pan on the trivet.
9. Lock the lid. Select Manual mode and set cooking time for 20 minutes on High Pressure.
10. When cooking is complete, allow the pressure to release naturally for 10 minutes and then release the remaining pressure. Allow the pie to rest in the pot for 5 minutes.
11. Preheat the oven broiler to 450°F (235°C).
12. Open the lid, remove the pan from the pot. Remove the foil and sprinkle the Cheddar over top of the pie.
13. Place the pie in the oven and broil for 2 minutes or until the cheese is melted and the top becomes golden brown. Slice into six equal-sized wedges. Serve hot.

Per Serving

calories: 225 | fat: 14.3g | protein: 22.0g | carbs: 2.5g | net carbs: 1.3g | fiber: 1.2g

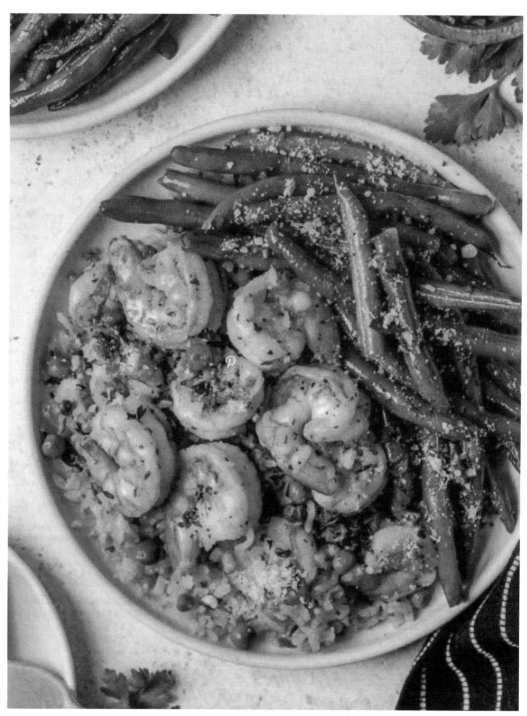

CHAPTER 7
Fish and Seafood

Stir-Fry Shrimp and Cauliflower

Prep time: 3 minutes | Cook time: 10 minutes | Serves 2

- 1 pound (454 g) shrimp, peeled and deveined
- ½ teaspoon salt
- ¼ teaspoon pepper
- ¼ teaspoon dried parsley
- ¼ teaspoon garlic powder
- 6 asparagus spears, cut into bite-sized pieces
- 1 cup water
- 2 tablespoons butter
- 1 cup uncooked cauliflower rice

1. Sprinkle seasoning on shrimp and place in a steamer basket. Add the asparagus to the basket.
2. Pour water into Instant Pot and insert the steamer basket.
3. Lock the lid. Select the Steam mode and set the cooking time for 5 minutes at Low Pressure.
4. Once cooking is complete, do a quick pressure release. Carefully open the lid.
5. Remove steamer basket and pour water out of Instant Pot.
6. Press the Sauté button on the Instant Pot and melt the butter.
7. Add the cauliflower rice and cooked shrimp and asparagus. Stir-fry for 3 to 5 minutes until cauliflower is tender.
8. Serve warm.

Per Serving

calories: 286 | fat: 12.6g | protein: 33.3g | carbs: 6.2g | net carbs: 4.1g | fiber: 2.1g

Tuna Salad with Tomatoes and Peppers

Prep time: 10 minutes | Cook time: 4 minutes | Serves 4

- 1½ cups water
- 1 pound (454 g) tuna steaks
- 1 green bell pepper, sliced
- 1 red bell pepper, sliced
- 2 Roma tomatoes, sliced
- 1 head lettuce
- 1 red onion, chopped
- 2 tablespoons Kalamata olives, pitted and halved
- 2 tablespoons extra-virgin olive oil
- 2 tablespoons balsamic vinegar
- ½ teaspoon chili flakes
- Sea salt, to taste

1. Add the water to the Instant Pot and insert a steamer basket.
2. Arrange the tuna steaks in the basket. Put the bell peppers and tomato slices on top.
3. Lock the lid. Select the Manual mode and set the cooking time for 4 minutes at High Pressure.
4. When the timer beeps, perform a quick pressure release. Carefully remove the lid.
5. Flake the fish with a fork.
6. Divide the lettuce leaves among 4 serving plates to make a bed for your salad. Add the onion and olives. Drizzle with the olive oil and balsamic vinegar.
7. Season with the chili flakes and salt. Place the prepared fish, tomatoes, and bell peppers on top.
8. Serve immediately.

Per Serving

calories: 170 | fat: 4.8g | protein: 23.9g | carbs: 7.6g | net carbs: 6.0g | fiber: 1.6g

Cheesy Trout Casserole

Prep time: 5 minutes | Cook time: 10 minutes | Serves 3

- 1½ cups water
- 1½ tablespoons olive oil
- 3 plum tomatoes, sliced
- ½ teaspoon dried oregano
- 1 teaspoon dried basil
- 3 trout fillets
- ½ teaspoon cayenne pepper, or more to taste
- ⅓ teaspoon black pepper
- Salt, to taste
- 1 bay leaf
- 1 cup shredded Pepper-Jack cheese

1. Pour the water into your Instant Pot and insert a trivet.
2. Grease a baking dish with the olive oil. Add the tomatoes slices to the baking dish and sprinkle with the oregano and basil.
3. Add the fish fillets and season with the cayenne pepper, black pepper, and salt. Add the bay leaf. Lower the baking dish onto the trivet.
4. Lock the lid. Select the Manual mode and set the cooking time for 10 minutes at High Pressure.
5. When the timer beeps, perform a quick pressure release. Carefully remove the lid.
6. Scatter the Pepper-Jack cheese on top, lock the lid, and allow the cheese to melt.
7. Serve warm.

Per Serving
calories: 361 | fat: 23.5g | protein: 25.2g | carbs: 12.1g | net carbs: 11.3g | fiber: 0.8g

Rainbow Trout with Mixed Greens

Prep time: 5 minutes | Cook time: 12 minutes | Serves 4

- 1 cup water
- 1½ (680 g) pounds rainbow trout fillets
- 4 tablespoons melted butter, divided
- Sea salt and ground black pepper, to taste
- 1 pound (454 g) mixed greens, trimmed
- and torn into pieces
- 1 bunch of scallions
- ½ cup chicken broth
- 1 tablespoon apple cider vinegar
- 1 teaspoon cayenne pepper

1. Pour the water into your Instant Pot and insert a steamer basket.
2. Add the fish to the basket. Drizzle with 1 tablespoon of the melted butter and season with the salt and black pepper.
3. Lock the lid. Select the Manual mode and set the cooking time for 12 minutes at Low pressure.
4. When the timer beeps, perform a quick pressure release. Carefully remove the lid.
5. Wipe down the Instant Pot with a damp cloth.
6. Add and warm the remaining 3 tablespoons of butter. Once hot, add the greens, scallions, broth, vinegar, and cayenne pepper and cook until the greens are wilted, stirring occasionally.
7. Serve the prepared trout fillets with the greens on the side.

Per Serving
calories: 349 | fat: 18.1g | protein: 38.9g | carbs: 7.7g | net carbs: 3.3g | fiber: 4.4g

Cheesy Fish Bake with Veggies

Prep time: 10 minutes | Cook time: 5 minutes | Serves 4

- 1½ cups water
- Cooking spray
- 2 ripe tomatoes, sliced
- 2 cloves garlic, minced
- 1 teaspoon dried oregano
- 1 teaspoon dried basil
- ½ teaspoon dried rosemary
- 1 red onion, sliced
- 1 head cauliflower, cut into florets
- 1 pound (454 g) tilapia fillets, sliced
- Sea salt, to taste
- 1 tablespoon olive oil
- 1 cup crumbled feta cheese
- ⅓ cup Kalamata olives, pitted and halved

1. Pour the water into your Instant Pot and insert a trivet.
2. Spritz a casserole dish with cooking spray. Add the tomato slices to the dish. Scatter the top with the garlic, oregano, basil, and rosemary.
3. Mix in the onion and cauliflower. Arrange the fish fillets on top. Sprinkle with the salt and drizzle with the olive oil.
4. Place the feta cheese and Kalamata olives on top. Lower the dish onto the trivet.
5. Lock the lid. Select the Manual mode and set the cooking time for 5 minutes at High Pressure.
6. When the timer beeps, perform a quick pressure release. Carefully remove the lid.
7. Allow to cool for 5 minutes before serving.

Per Serving

calories: 302 | fat: 15.0g | protein: 30.5g | carbs: 11.3g | net carbs: 8.2g | fiber: 3.1g

Halibut Stew with Bacon and Cheese

Prep time: 10 minutes | Cook time: 10 minutes | Serves 4

- 4 slices bacon, chopped
- 1 celery, chopped
- ½ cup chopped shallots
- 1 teaspoon garlic, smashed
- 1 pound (454 g) halibut
- 2 cups fish stock
- 1 tablespoon coconut oil, softened
- ¼ teaspoon ground allspice
- Sea salt and crushed black peppercorns, to taste
- 1 cup Cottage cheese, at room temperature
- 1 cup heavy cream

1. Set the Instant Pot to Sauté. Cook the bacon until crispy.
2. Add the celery, shallots, and garlic and sauté for another 2 minutes, or until the vegetables are just tender.
3. Mix in the halibut, stock, coconut oil, allspice, salt, and black peppercorns. Stir well.
4. Lock the lid. Select the Manual mode and set the cooking time for 7 minutes at Low Pressure.
5. When the timer beeps, perform a natural pressure release for 10 minutes, then release any remaining pressure. Carefully remove the lid.
6. Stir in the cheese and heavy cream. Select the Sauté mode again and let it simmer for a few minutes until heated through.
7. Serve immediately.

Per Serving

calories: 531 | fat: 43.6g | protein: 29.1g | carbs: 5.7g | net carbs: 5.1g | fiber: 0.6g

Lemony Mahi-Mahi fillets with Peppers

Prep time: 10 minutes | Cook time: 3 minutes | Serves 3

- 2 sprigs fresh rosemary
- 2 sprigs dill, tarragon
- 1 sprig fresh thyme
- 1 cup water
- 1 lemon, sliced
- 3 mahi-mahi fillets

- 2 tablespoons coconut oil, melted
- Sea salt and ground black pepper, to taste
- 1 serrano pepper, seeded and sliced
- 1 green bell pepper, sliced
- 1 red bell pepper, sliced

1. Add the herbs, water, and lemon slices to the Instant Pot and insert a steamer basket.
2. Arrange the mahi-mahi fillets in the steamer basket.
3. Drizzle the melted coconut oil over the top and season with the salt and black pepper.
4. Lock the lid. Select the Manual mode and set the cooking time for 3 minutes at Low Pressure.
5. When the timer beeps, perform a natural pressure release for 10 minutes, then release any remaining pressure. Carefully remove the lid.
6. Place the peppers on top. Select the Sauté mode and let it simmer for another 1 minute.
7. Serve immediately.

Per Serving

calories: 454 | fat: 14.7g | protein: 76.4g | carbs: 4.1g | net carbs: 3.5g | fiber: 0.6g

Snapper in Spicy Tomato Sauce

Prep time: 5 minutes | Cook time: 5 minutes | Serves 6

- 2 teaspoons coconut oil, melted
- 1 teaspoon celery seeds
- ½ teaspoon fresh grated ginger
- ½ teaspoon cumin seeds
- 1 yellow onion, chopped
- 2 cloves garlic, minced
- 1½ pounds (680 g) snapper fillets
- ¾ cup vegetable broth

- 1 (14-ounce / 113-g) can fire-roasted diced tomatoes
- 1 bell pepper, sliced
- 1 jalapeño pepper, minced
- Sea salt and ground black pepper, to taste
- ¼ teaspoon chili flakes
- ½ teaspoon turmeric powder

1. Set the Instant Pot to Sauté. Add and heat the sesame oil until hot. Sauté the celery seeds, fresh ginger, and cumin seeds.
2. Add the onion and continue to sauté until softened and fragrant.
3. Mix in the minced garlic and continue to cook for 30 seconds. Add the remaining ingredients and stir well.
4. Lock the lid. Select the Manual mode and set the cooking time for 3 minutes at Low Pressure.
5. When the timer beeps, perform a quick pressure release. Carefully remove the lid.
6. Serve warm

Per Serving

calories: 177 | fat: 5.9g | protein: 25.8g | carbs: 5.1g | net carbs: 3.7g | fiber: 1.4g

Aromatic Monkfish Stew

Prep time: 5 minutes | Cook time: 6 minutes | Serves 6

- Juice of 1 lemon
- 1 tablespoon fresh basil
- 1 tablespoon fresh parsley
- 1 tablespoon olive oil
- 1 teaspoon garlic, minced
- 1½ pounds (680 g) monkfish
- 1 tablespoon butter
- 1 bell pepper, chopped
- 1 onion, sliced
- ½ teaspoon cayenne pepper
- ½ teaspoon mixed peppercorns
- ¼ teaspoon turmeric powder
- ¼ teaspoon ground cumin
- Sea salt and ground black pepper, to taste
- 2 cups fish stock
- ½ cup water
- ¼ cup dry white wine
- 2 bay leaves
- 1 ripe tomato, crushed

1. Stir together the lemon juice, basil, parsley, olive oil, and garlic in a ceramic dish. Add the monkfish and marinate for 30 minutes.
2. Set your Instant Pot to Sauté. Add and melt the butter. Once hot, cook the bell pepper and onion until fragrant.
3. Stir in the remaining ingredients.
4. Lock the lid. Select the Manual mode and set the cooking time for 6 minutes at High Pressure.
5. When the timer beeps, perform a quick pressure release. Carefully remove the lid.
6. Discard the bay leaves and divide your stew into serving bowls.
7. Serve hot.

Per Serving

calories: 153 | fat: 6.9g | protein: 18.9g | carbs: 3.8g | net carbs: 3.0g | fiber: 0.8g

Haddock and Veggie Foil Packets

Prep time: 5 minutes | Cook time: 10 minutes | Serves 4

- 1½ cups water
- 1 lemon, sliced
- 2 bell peppers, sliced
- 1 brown onion, sliced into rings
- 4 sprigs parsley
- 2 sprigs thyme
- 2 sprigs rosemary
- 4 haddock fillets
- Sea salt, to taste
- ⅓ teaspoon ground black pepper, or more to taste
- 2 tablespoons extra-virgin olive oil

1. Pour the water and lemon into your Instant Pot and insert a steamer basket.
2. Assemble the packets with large sheets of heavy-duty foil.
3. Place the peppers, onion rings, parsley, thyme, and rosemary in the center of each foil. Place the fish fillets on top of the veggies.
4. Sprinkle with the salt and black pepper and drizzle the olive oil over the fillets. Place the packets in the steamer basket.
5. Lock the lid. Select the Manual mode and set the cooking time for 10 minutes at Low Pressure.
6. When the timer beeps, perform a quick pressure release. Carefully remove the lid.
7. Serve warm.

Per Serving

calories: 218 | fat: 7.7g | protein: 32.3g | carbs: 4.8g | net carbs: 4.0g | fiber: 0.8g

Lemony Fish and Asparagus

Prep time: 5 minutes | Cook time: 3 minutes | Serves 4

- 2 lemons
- 2 cups cold water
- 2 tablespoons extra-virgin olive oil
- 4 (4-ounce / 113-g) white fish fillets, such as cod or haddock
- 1 teaspoon fine sea salt
- 1 teaspoon ground black pepper
- 1 bundle asparagus, ends trimmed
- 2 tablespoons lemon juice
- Fresh dill, for garnish

1. Grate the zest off the lemons until you have about 1 tablespoon and set the zest aside. Slice the lemons into ⅛-inch slices.
2. Pour the water into the Instant Pot. Add 1 tablespoon of the olive oil to each of two stackable steamer pans.
3. Sprinkle the fish on all sides with the lemon zest, salt, and pepper.
4. Arrange two fillets in each steamer pan and top each with the lemon slices and then the asparagus. Sprinkle the asparagus with the salt and drizzle the lemon juice over the top.
5. Stack the steamer pans in the Instant Pot. Cover the top steamer pan with its lid.
6. Lock the lid. Select the Manual mode and set the cooking time for 3 minutes at High Pressure.
7. Once cooking is complete, do a natural pressure release for 7 minutes, then release any remaining pressure. Carefully open the lid.
8. Lift the steamer pans out of the Instant Pot.
9. Transfer the fish and asparagus to a serving plate. Garnish with the lemon slices and dill.
10. Serve immediately.

Per Serving
calories: 163 | fat: 5.8g | protein: 23.7g | carbs: 7.1g | net carbs: 4.1g | fiber: 3.0g

Spicy Shrimp Salad

Prep time: 5 minutes | Cook time: 7 minutes | Serves 2

- 1 pound (454 g) shrimp, peeled and deveined
- ½ teaspoon Old Bay seasoning
- ¼ teaspoon pepper
- ¼ teaspoon salt
- ⅛ teaspoon cayenne
- ⅛ teaspoon garlic powder
- 1 cup water
- ¼ cup mayonnaise
- 2 tablespoons chili paste

1. Toss shrimp in a 7-cup glass bowl with Old Bay seasoning, salt, pepper, cayenne, and garlic powder.
2. Pour the water into Instant Pot and insert the trivet. Place the bowl with shrimp on top.
3. Lock the lid. Select the Steam mode and set the cooking time for 7 minutes at Low Pressure.
4. Once cooking is complete, do a quick pressure release. Carefully open the lid.
5. Remove the bowl from the Instant Pot and drain water.
6. In a small bowl, stir together the mayo and chili paste. Add the shrimp and toss to coat. Serve immediately.

Per Serving
calories: 403 | fat: 24.7g | protein: 32.9g | carbs: 8.3g | net carbs: 8.2g | fiber: 0.1g

Fish Packets with Pesto and Cheese

Prep time: 8 minutes | Cook time: 6 minutes | Serves 4

- ✿ 1½ cups cold water.
- ✿ 4 (4-ounce / 113-g) white fish fillets, such as cod or haddock
- ✿ 1 teaspoon fine sea salt
- ✿ ½ teaspoon ground black pepper
- ✿ 1 (4-ounce / 113-g) jar pesto
- ✿ ½ cup shredded Parmesan cheese (about 2 ounces / 57 g)
- ✿ Halved cherry tomatoes, for garnish

1. Pour the water into your Instant Pot and insert a steamer basket.
2. Sprinkle the fish on all sides with the salt and pepper. Take four sheets of parchment paper and place a fillet in the center of each sheet.
3. Dollop 2 tablespoons of the pesto on top of each fillet and sprinkle with 2 tablespoons of the Parmesan cheese.
4. Wrap the fish in the parchment by folding in the edges and folding down the top like an envelope to close tightly.
5. Stack the packets in the steamer basket, seam-side down.
6. Lock the lid. Select the Manual mode and set the cooking time for 6 minutes at Low Pressure.
7. Once cooking is complete, do a natural pressure release for 10 minutes, then release any remaining pressure. Carefully open the lid.
8. Remove the fish packets from the pot. Transfer to a serving plate and garnish with the cherry tomatoes.
9. Serve immediately.

Per Serving

calories: 257 | fat: 17.8g | protein: 23.7g | carbs: 2.3g | net carbs: 1.3g | fiber: 1.0g

Smoked Sausage and Grouper

Prep time: 5 minutes | Cook time: 10 minutes | Serves 4

- ✿ 2 tablespoons butter
- ✿ ½ pound (227 g) smoked turkey sausage, casing removed
- ✿ 1 pound (454 g) cremini mushrooms, sliced
- ✿ 2 garlic cloves, minced
- ✿ 4 grouper fillets
- ✿ ½ cup dry white wine
- ✿ Sea salt, to taste
- ✿ ½ teaspoon freshly cracked black peppercorns
- ✿ 1 tablespoon fresh lime juice
- ✿ 2 tablespoons chopped fresh cilantro

1. Set your Instant Pot to Sauté and melt the butter.
2. Add the sausage and cook until nicely browned on all sides. Remove the sausage and set aside.
3. Add the mushrooms and cook for about 3 minutes or until fragrant.
4. Add the garlic and continue to sauté for another 30 seconds.
5. Add the fish, wine, salt, and black peppercorns. Return the sausage to the Instant Pot.
6. Lock the lid. Select the Manual mode and set the cooking time for 3 minutes at Low Pressure.
7. When the timer beeps, perform a quick pressure release. Carefully remove the lid.
8. Drizzle with the lime juice and serve garnished with fresh cilantro.

Per Serving

calories: 409 | fat: 13.5g | protein: 61.9g | carbs: 8.7g | net carbs: 7.4g | fiber: 1.3g

Cod Fillets with Cherry Tomatoes

Prep time: 2 minutes | Cook time: 15 minutes | Serves 4

- 2 tablespoons butter
- ¼ cup diced onion
- 1 clove garlic, minced
- 1 cup cherry tomatoes, halved
- ¼ cup chicken broth
- ¼ teaspoon dried thyme
- ¼ teaspoon salt
- ⅛ teaspoon pepper
- 4 (4-ounce / 113-g) cod fillets
- 1 cup water
- ¼ cup fresh chopped Italian parsley

1. Set your Instant Pot to Sauté. Add and melt the butter. Once hot, add the onions and cook until softened. Add the garlic and cook for another 30 seconds.
2. Add the tomatoes, chicken broth, thyme, salt, and pepper. Continue to cook for 5 to 7 minutes, or until the tomatoes start to soften.
3. Pour the sauce into a glass bowl. Add the fish fillets. Cover with foil.
4. Pour the water into the Instant Pot and insert a trivet. Place the bowl on top.
5. Lock the lid. Select the Manual mode and set the cooking time for 3 minutes at Low Pressure.
6. Once cooking is complete, do a quick pressure release. Carefully open the lid.
7. Sprinkle with the fresh parsley and serve.

Per Serving

calories: 159 | fat: 7.9g | protein: 21.7g | carbs: 3.0g | net carbs: 2.1g| fiber: 0.9g

Swai with Port Wine Sauce

Prep time: 5 minutes | Cook time: 10 minutes | Serves 4

- 1 tablespoon butter
- 1 teaspoon fresh grated ginger
- 2 garlic cloves, minced
- 2 tablespoon chopped green onions
- 1 pound (454 g) swai fish fillets
- ½ cup port wine
- 1 teaspoon parsley flakes
- ½ tablespoon lemon juice
- ½ teaspoon chili flakes
- ½ teaspoon cayenne pepper
- ½ teaspoon fennel seeds
- ¼ teaspoon ground bay leaf
- Coarse sea salt and ground black pepper, to taste

1. Set your Instant Pot to Sauté and melt the butter.
2. Cook the ginger, garlic, and green onions for 2 minutes until softened. Add the remaining ingredients and gently stir to incorporate.
3. Lock the lid. Select the Manual mode and set the cooking time for 6 minutes at Low Pressure.
4. When the timer beeps, perform a quick pressure release. Carefully remove the lid.
5. Serve warm.

Per Serving

calories: 112 | fat: 3.5g | protein: 17.8g | carbs: 1.7g | net carbs: 1.3g | fiber: 0.4g

Garam Masala Fish

Prep time: 10 minutes | Cook time: 10 minutes | Serves 4

- ✿ 2 tablespoons sesame oil
- ✿ ½ teaspoon cumin seeds
- ✿ ½ cup chopped leeks
- ✿ 1 teaspoon ginger-garlic paste
- ✿ 1 pound (454 g) cod fillets, boneless and sliced
- ✿ 2 ripe tomatoes, chopped
- ✿ 1½ tablespoons fresh lemon juice
- ✿ ½ teaspoon garam masala
- ✿ ½ teaspoon turmeric powder
- ✿ 1 tablespoon chopped fresh dill leaves
- ✿ 1 tablespoon chopped fresh curry leaves
- ✿ 1 tablespoon chopped fresh parsley leaves
- ✿ Coarse sea salt, to taste
- ✿ ½ teaspoon smoked cayenne pepper
- ✿ ¼ teaspoon ground black pepper, or more to taste

1. Set the Instant Pot to Sauté. Add and heat the sesame oil until hot. Sauté the cumin seeds for 30 seconds.
2. Add the leeks and cook for another 2 minutes until translucent. Add the ginger-garlic paste and cook for an additional 40 seconds.
3. Stir in the remaining ingredients.
4. Lock the lid. Select the Manual mode and set the cooking time for 6 minutes at Low Pressure.
5. When the timer beeps, perform a quick pressure release. Carefully remove the lid.
6. Serve immediately.

Per Serving
calories: 166 | fat: 7.8g | protein: 18.4g | carbs: 5.9g | net carbs: 3.9g | fiber: 2.0g

Garlic Tuna Casserole

Prep time: 7 minutes | Cook time: 9 minutes | Serves 4

- ✿ 1 cup grated Parmesan or shredded Cheddar cheese, plus more for topping
- ✿ 1 (8-ounce / 227-g) package cream cheese (1 cup), softened
- ✿ ½ cup chicken broth
- ✿ 1 tablespoon unsalted butter
- ✿ ½ small head cauliflower, cut into 1-inch pieces
- ✿ 1 cup diced onions
- ✿ 2 cloves garlic, minced, or more to taste
- ✿ 2 (4-ounce / 113-g) cans chunk tuna packed in water, drained
- ✿ 1½ cups cold water

For Garnish:
- ✿ Chopped fresh flat-leaf parsley
- ✿ Sliced green onions
- ✿ Cherry tomatoes, halved
- ✿ Ground black pepper

1. In a blender, add the Parmesan cheese, cream cheese, and broth and blitz until smooth. Set aside.
2. Set your Instant Pot to Sauté. Add and melt the butter. Add the cauliflower and onions and sauté for 4 minutes, or until the onions are softened. Fold in the garlic and sauté for an additional 1 minute.
3. Place the cheese sauce and tuna in a large bowl. Mix in the veggies and stir well. Transfer the mixture to a casserole dish.
4. Place a trivet in the bottom of your Instant Pot and add the cold water. Use a foil sling, lower the casserole dish onto the trivet. Tuck in the sides of the sling.
5. Lock the lid. Select the Manual mode and set the cooking time for 5 minutes for al dente cauliflower or 8 minutes for softer cauliflower at High Pressure.
6. Once cooking is complete, do a quick pressure release. Carefully open the lid.
7. Serve topped with the cheese and garnished with the parsley, green onions, cherry tomatoes, and freshly ground pepper.

Per Serving
calories: 378 | fat: 26.8g | protein: 23.8g | carbs: 10.5g | net carbs: 9.3g | fiber: 1.2g

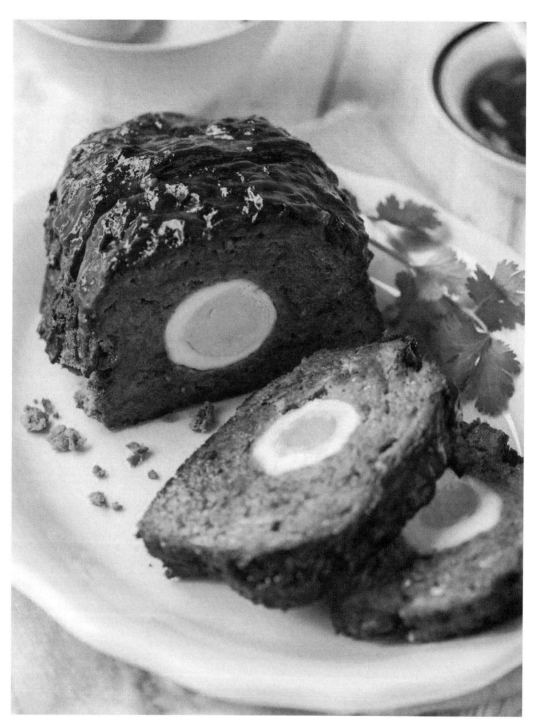

CHAPTER 8
Pork

Egg Meatloaf

Prep time: 20 minutes | Cook time: 25 minutes | Serves 6

- ✿ 1 tablespoon avocado oil
- ✿ 1½ cup ground pork
- ✿ 1 teaspoon chives
- ✿ 1 teaspoon salt
- ✿ ½ teaspoon ground black pepper
- ✿ 2 tablespoons coconut flour
- ✿ 3 eggs, hard-boiled, peeled
- ✿ 1 cup water

1. Brush a loaf pan with avocado oil.
2. In the mixing bowl, mix the ground pork, chives, salt, ground black pepper, and coconut flour.
3. Transfer the mixture in the loaf pan and flatten with a spatula.
4. Fill the meatloaf with hard-boiled eggs.
5. Pour water and insert the trivet in the Instant Pot.
6. Lower the loaf pan over the trivet in the Instant Pot. Close the lid.
7. Select Manual mode and set cooking time for 25 minutes on High Pressure.
8. When timer beeps, use a natural pressure release for 10 minutes, then release any remaining pressure. Open the lid.
9. Serve immediately.

Per Serving

calories: 277 | fat: 19.0g | protein: 23.3g | carbs: 2.1g | net carbs: 0.9g | fiber: 1.2g

Albóndigas Sinaloenses

Prep time: 15 minutes | Cook time: 10 minutes | Serves 6

- ✿ 1 pound (454 g) ground pork
- ✿ ½ pound (227 g) Italian sausage, crumbled
- ✿ 2 tablespoons yellow onion, finely chopped
- ✿ ½ teaspoon dried oregano
- ✿ 1 sprig fresh mint, finely minced
- ✿ ½ teaspoon ground cumin
- ✿ 2 garlic cloves, finely minced
- ✿ ¼ teaspoon fresh ginger, grated
- ✿ Seasoned salt and ground black pepper, to taste
- ✿ 1 tablespoon olive oil
- ✿ ½ cup yellow onions, finely chopped
- ✿ 2 chipotle chilies in adobo
- ✿ 2 tomatoes, puréed
- ✿ 2 tablespoons tomato passata
- ✿ 1 cup chicken broth

1. In a mixing bowl, combine the pork, sausage, 2 tablespoons of yellow onion, oregano, mint, cumin, garlic, ginger, salt, and black pepper.
2. Roll the mixture into meatballs and reserve.
3. Press the Sauté button to heat up the Instant Pot. Heat the olive oil and cook the meatballs for 4 minutes, stirring continuously.
4. Stir in ½ cup of yellow onions, chilies in adobo, tomatoes passata, and broth. Add reserved meatballs.
5. Secure the lid. Choose the Manual mode and set cooking time for 6 minutes at High pressure.
6. Once cooking is complete, use a quick pressure release. Carefully remove the lid.
7. Serve immediately.

Per Serving

calories: 408 | fat: 31.1g | protein: 26.5g | carbs: 4.7g | net carbs: 2.4g | fiber: 2.3g

Aromatic Pork Steak Curry

Prep time: 15 minutes | Cook time: 8 minutes | Serves 6

- ½ teaspoon mustard seeds
- 1 teaspoon fennel seeds
- 1 teaspoon cumin seeds
- 2 chili peppers, deseeded and minced
- ½ teaspoon ground bay leaf
- 1 teaspoon mixed peppercorns
- 1 tablespoon sesame oil
- 1½ pounds (680 g) pork steak, sliced
- 2 cloves garlic, finely minced
- 2 tablespoons scallions, chopped
- 1 teaspoon fresh ginger, grated
- 1 teaspoon curry powder
- 1 cup chicken broth
- 2 tablespoons balsamic vinegar
- 3 tablespoons coconut cream
- ¼ teaspoon red pepper flakes, crushed
- Sea salt, to taste
- ¼ teaspoon ground black pepper

1. Heat a skillet over medium-high heat. Once hot, roast the mustard seeds, fennel seeds, cumin seeds, chili peppers, ground bay leaf, and peppercorns for 1 or 2 minutes or until aromatic.
2. Press the Sauté button to heat up the Instant Pot. Heat the sesame oil until sizzling. Sear pork steak for 5 minutes or until browned.
3. Add the remaining ingredients, including roasted seasonings. Stir to mix well.
4. Secure the lid. Choose the Manual mode and set cooking time for 8 minutes on High pressure.
5. Once cooking is complete, use a quick pressure release. Carefully remove the lid.
6. Serve immediately.

Per Serving

calories: 362 | fat: 25.2g | protein: 29.6g | carbs: 2.2g | net carbs: 0.9g | fiber: 1.3g

---

Bacon-Wrapped Pork Bites

Prep time: 15 minutes | Cook time: 20 minutes | Serves 4

- 3 tablespoons butter
- 10 ounces (283 g) pork tenderloin, cubed
- 6 ounces (170 g) bacon, sliced
- ½ teaspoon white pepper
- ¾ cup chicken stock

1. Melt the butter on Sauté mode in the Instant Pot.
2. Meanwhile, wrap the pork tenderloin cubes in the sliced bacon and sprinkle with white pepper. Secure with toothpicks, if necessary.
3. Put the wrapped pork tenderloin in the melted butter and cook for 3 minutes on each side.
4. Add the chicken stock and close the lid.
5. Select Manual mode and set cooking time for 14 minutes on High Pressure.
6. When timer beeps, use a natural pressure release for 5 minutes, then release any remaining pressure. Open the lid.
7. Discard the toothpicks and serve immediately.

Per Serving

calories: 410 | fat: 29.0g | protein: 34.6g | carbs: 0.9g | net carbs: 0.8g | fiber: 0.1g

Beery Boston-Style Butt

Prep time: 10 minutes | Cook time: 1 hour 1 minutes | Serves 4

- ✿ 1 tablespoon butter
- ✿ 1 pound (454 g) Boston-style butt
- ✿ ½ cup leeks, chopped
- ✿ ¼ cup beer
- ✿ ½ cup chicken stock
- ✿ Pinch of grated nutmeg
- ✿ Sea salt, to taste
- ✿ ¼ teaspoon ground black pepper
- ✿ ¼ cup water

1. Press the Sauté button to heat up the Instant Pot. Once hot, melt the butter.
2. Cook the Boston-style butt for 3 minutes on each side. Remove from the pot and reserve.
3. Sauté the leeks for 5 minutes or until fragrant. Add the remaining ingredients and stir to combine.
4. Secure the lid. Choose the Manual mode and set cooking time for 50 minutes on High pressure.
5. Once cooking is complete, use a natural pressure release for 20 minutes, then release any remaining pressure. Carefully remove the lid.
6. Serve immediately.

Per Serving

calories: 330 | fat: 13.1g | protein: 48.4g | carbs: 2.1g | net carbs: 0.4g | fiber: 1.7g

Blade Pork with Sauerkraut

Prep time: 15 minutes | Cook time: 37 minutes | Serves 6

- ✿ 2 pounds (907 g) blade pork steaks
- ✿ Sea salt and ground black pepper, to taste
- ✿ ½ teaspoon cayenne pepper
- ✿ ½ teaspoon dried parsley flakes
- ✿ 1 tablespoon butter
- ✿ 1½ cups water
- ✿ 2 cloves garlic, thinly sliced
- ✿ 2 pork sausages, casing removed and sliced
- ✿ 4 cups sauerkraut

1. Season the blade pork steaks with salt, black pepper, cayenne pepper, and dried parsley.
2. Press the Sauté button to heat up the Instant Pot. Melt the butter and sear blade pork steaks for 5 minutes or until browned on all sides.
3. Clean the Instant Pot. Add water and trivet to the bottom of the Instant Pot.
4. Place the blade pork steaks on the trivet. Make small slits over entire pork with a knife. Insert garlic pieces into each slit.
5. Secure the lid. Choose the Meat/Stew mode and set cooking time for 30 minutes on High pressure.
6. Once cooking is complete, use a natural pressure release for 15 minutes, then release any remaining pressure. Carefully remove the lid.
7. Add the sausage and sauerkraut. Press the Sauté button and cook for 2 minutes more or until heated through.
8. Serve immediately.

Per Serving

calories: 471 | fat: 27.3g | protein: 47.7g | carbs: 8.4g | net carbs: 2.0g | fiber: 6.4g

Bo Ssäm

Prep time: 10 minutes | Cook time: 8 minutes | Serves 6

- 1 tablespoon vegetable oil
- 1 pound (454 g) ground pork
- 2 tablespoons gochujang
- 1 tablespoon Doubanjiang
- ½ teaspoon ground Sichuan peppercorns
- 1 tablespoon minced fresh ginger
- 1 tablespoon minced garlic
- 1 tablespoon coconut aminos
- 1 teaspoon hot sesame oil
- 1 teaspoon salt
- ¼ cup water
- 1 bunch bok choy, chopped (about 4 to 6 cups)

1. Preheat the Instant Pot on Sauté mode. Add the oil and heat until it is shimmering.
2. Add the ground pork, breaking up all lumps, and cook for 4 minutes or until the pork is no longer pink.
3. Add the gochujang, doubanjiang, peppercorns, ginger, garlic, coconut aminos, sesame oil, and salt. Stir to combine.
4. Add the water and bok choy.
5. Lock the lid. Select Manual mode. Set cooking time for 4 minutes on High Pressure.
6. When cooking is complete, quick-release the pressure. Unlock the lid.
7. Serve immediately.

Per Serving
calories: 239 | fat: 19.0g | protein: 14.0g | carbs: 2.0g | net carbs: 1.0g | fiber: 1.0g

Easy Ginger Pork Meatballs

Prep time: 10 minutes | Cook time: 7 minutes | Serves 3

- 11 ounces (312 g) ground pork
- 1 teaspoon ginger paste
- 1 teaspoon lemon juice
- ¼ teaspoon chili flakes
- 1 tablespoon butter
- ¼ cup water

1. Combine the ground pork and ginger paste in a large bowl.
2. Mix in the lemon juice and chili flakes.
3. Put the butter in the Instant Pot and melt on Sauté mode.
4. Meanwhile, shape the mixture into small meatballs.
5. Place the meatballs in the Instant Pot and cook for 2 minutes on each side.
6. Add water and lock the lid.
7. Set the Manual mode and set cooking time for 3 minutes on High Pressure.
8. When timer beeps, perform a quick pressure release. Open the lid.
9. Serve warm.

Per Serving
calories: 278 | fat: 11.3g | protein: 41.0g | carbs: 0.7g | net carbs: 0.6g | fiber: 0.1g

Coconut Pork Muffins

Prep time: 5 minutes | Cook time: 9 minutes | Serves 2

- 1 egg, beaten
- 2 tablespoons coconut flour
- 1 teaspoon parsley
- ¼ teaspoon salt
- 1 tablespoon coconut cream
- 4 ounces (113 g) ground pork, fried
- 1 cup water

1. Whisk together the egg, coconut flour, parsley, salt, and coconut cream. Add the fried ground pork. Mix the the mixture until homogenous.
2. Pour the mixture into a muffin pan.
3. Pour the water in the Instant Pot and place in the trivet.
4. Lower the muffin pan on the trivet and close the Instant Pot lid.
5. Set the Manual mode and set cooking time for 4 minutes on High Pressure.
6. When timer beeps, perform a natural pressure release for 5 minutes, then release any remaining pressure. Open the lid.
7. Serve warm.

Per Serving

calories: 160 | fat: 6.7g | protein: 18.8g | carbs: 5.6g | net carbs: 2.4g | fiber: 3.2g

Easy Pork Steaks with Pico de Gallo

Prep time: 15 minutes | Cook time: 12 minutes | Serves 6

- 1 tablespoon butter
- 2 pounds (907 g) pork steaks
- 1 bell pepper, deseeded and sliced
- ½ cup shallots, chopped
- 2 garlic cloves, minced
- ¼ cup dry red wine
- 1 cup chicken bone broth
- ¼ cup water
- Salt, to taste
- ¼ teaspoon freshly ground black pepper, or more to taste
- Pico de Gallo:
- 1 tomato, chopped
- 1 chili pepper, seeded and minced
- ½ cup red onion, chopped
- 2 garlic cloves, minced
- 1 tablespoon fresh cilantro, finely chopped
- Sea salt, to taste

1. Press the Sauté button to heat up the Instant Pot. Melt the butter and sear the pork steaks about 4 minutes or until browned on both sides.
2. Add bell pepper, shallot, garlic, wine, chicken bone broth, water, salt, and black pepper to the Instant Pot.
3. Secure the lid. Choose the Manual mode and set cooking time for 8 minutes at High pressure.
4. Meanwhile, combine the ingredients for the Pico de Gallo in a small bowl. Refrigerate until ready to serve.
5. Once cooking is complete, use a quick pressure release. Carefully remove the lid.
6. Serve warm pork steaks with the chilled Pico de Gallo on the side.

Per Serving

calories: 448 | fat: 29.2g | protein: 39.4g | carbs: 4.1g | net carbs: 1.8g | fiber: 2.3g

Eggplant Pork Lasagna

Prep time: 20 minutes | Cook time: 30 minutes | Serves 6

- 2 eggplants, sliced
- 1 teaspoon salt
- 10 ounces (283 g) ground pork
- 1 cup Mozzarella, shredded
- 1 tablespoon unsweetened tomato purée
- 1 teaspoon butter, softened
- 1 cup chicken stock

1. Sprinkle the eggplants with salt and let sit for 10 minutes, then pat dry with paper towels.
2. In a mixing bowl, mix the ground pork, butter, and tomato purée.
3. Make a layer of the sliced eggplants in the bottom of the Instant Pot and top with ground pork mixture.
4. Top the ground pork with Mozzarella and repeat with remaining ingredients.
5. Pour in the chicken stock. Close the lid. Select Manual mode and set cooking time for 30 minutes on High Pressure.
6. When timer beeps, use a natural pressure release for 10 minutes, then release the remaining pressure and open the lid.
7. Cool for 10 minutes and serve.

Per Serving
calories: 136 | fat: 3.6g | protein: 15.7g | carbs: 11.5g | net carbs: 4.9g | fiber: 6.6g

Hawaiian Pulled Pork Roast with Cabbage

Prep time: 10 minutes | Cook time: 1 hour 2 minutes minutes | Serves 6

- 1½ tablespoons olive oil
- 3 pounds (1.4 kg) pork shoulder roast, cut into 4 equal-sized pieces
- 3 cloves garlic, minced
- 1 tablespoon liquid smoke
- 2 cups water, divided
- 1 tablespoon sea salt
- 2 cups shredded cabbage

1. Select Sauté mode and add the olive oil to the Instant Pot. Once the oil is hot, add the pork cuts and sear for 5 minutes per side or until browned. Once browned, transfer the pork to a platter and set aside.
2. Add the garlic, liquid smoke, and 1½ cups water to the Instant Pot. Stir to combine.
3. Return the pork to the pot and sprinkle the salt over top.
4. Lock the lid. Select Manual mode and set cooking time for 1 hour on High Pressure.
5. When cooking is complete, allow the pressure to release naturally for 20 minutes, then release any remaining pressure.
6. Open the lid and transfer the pork to a large platter. Using two forks, shred the pork. Set aside.
7. Add the shredded cabbage and remaining water to the liquid in the pot. Stir.
8. Lock the lid. Select Manual mode and set cooking time for 2 minutes on High Pressure. When cooking is complete, quick release the pressure.
9. Transfer the cabbage to the serving platter with the pork. Serve warm.

Per Serving
calories: 314 | fat: 12.0g | protein: 46.5g | carbs: 2.7g | net carbs: 2.0g | fiber: 0.7g

Hearty Barbecue Pork Ribs

Prep time: 6 minutes | Cook time: 35 minutes | Serves 5

- ✿ 1½ cups beef broth
- ✿ 2 pounds (907 g) country-style boneless pork ribs

For the Sauce:
- ✿ 1½ tablespoons unsalted butter
- ✿ ½ tablespoon Worcestershire sauce
- ✿ ½ teaspoon blackstrap molasses
- ✿ 1 cup unsweetened tomato purée
- ✿ 1 tablespoon apple cider vinegar

- ✿ 1½ teaspoons liquid smoke
- ✿ 2 tablespoons erythritol
- ✿ 1 teaspoon garlic powder
- ✿ ½ teaspoon sea salt
- ✿ ½ teaspoon onion powder

For the Dry Rub:
- ✿ 1½ teaspoons smoked paprika
- ✿ 1½ teaspoons onion powder
- ✿ 1 teaspoon garlic powder
- ✿ 1 teaspoon ground cumin

- ✿ 1 teaspoon sea salt
- ✿ 1 teaspoon ground black pepper
- ✿ ⅛ teaspoon cayenne pepper

1. Add the butter to a small saucepan and heat over medium heat.
2. Once the butter is melted, add the Worcestershire sauce, molasses, tomato purée, vinegar, liquid smoke, erythritol, garlic powder, sea salt, and onion powder. Stir until well combined and then remove from the heat. Set aside.
3. Comb the paprika, onion powder, garlic powder, cumin, sea salt, black pepper, and cayenne pepper in a small bowl. Mix well to combine. Set aside.
4. Add the beef broth to the Instant Pot and place the trivet in the pot.
5. Generously sprinkle the dry rub over the pork and gently rub the spices into the meat. Stack the seasoned ribs on the trivet.
6. Pour half the barbecue sauce over the ribs, reserving the remaining sauce for serving.
7. Lock the lid. Select Manual mode and set cooking time for 35 minutes on High Pressure.
8. When cooking is complete, allow the pressure to release naturally for 20 minutes, then release any remaining pressure.
9. Open the lid and use tongs to carefully transfer the ribs to a serving plate. Using a pastry brush, brush the reserved sauce over the ribs. Serve warm.

Per Serving

calories:398 | fat: 23.0g | protein: 36.0g | carbs: 11.8g | net carbs: 7.0g | fiber: 4.8g

Hearty Pork Carnitas

Prep time: 10 minutes | Cook time: 45 minutes | Serves 4

- 1 onion, sliced
- 4 garlic cloves, sliced
- 1 pound (454 g) pork shoulder, cut into cubes, visible fat removed
- Juice of 1 lemon
- ¼ teaspoon ancho chili powder
- ¼ teaspoon chipotle chili powder
- ½ teaspoon dried oregano
- ½ teaspoon roasted cumin powder
- ¼ teaspoon smoked paprika
- 1 to 2 teaspoons salt
- 1 teaspoon freshly ground black pepper
- ½ cup water
- 1 to 2 tablespoons coconut oil
- ½ cup sour cream
- ½ avocado, diced

1. Place the onion and garlic in the Instant Pot to help them release water when the meat is cooking.
2. In a large bowl, mix together the pork and lemon juice. Add the ancho chili powder, chipotle chili powder, oregano, cumin, paprika, salt, and pepper, and stir to combine.
3. Place the pork on top of the onions and garlic.
4. Pour the water into the bowl and swirl to get the last of the spices, then pour the liquid onto the pork.
5. Lock the lid. Select Meat/Stew mode. Set cooking time for 35 minutes on High Pressure.
6. When cooking is complete, let the pressure release naturally for 10 minutes, then release any remaining pressure. Unlock the lid.
7. Remove the pork, leaving the liquid in the pot.
8. Switch the pot to Sauté and bring the sauce to a boil until it is thickened.
9. Place a cast iron skillet over medium-high heat. Once it is hot, add the oil.
10. Shred the pork, then place in the skillet. Let the meat brown for 4 minutes.
11. When the meat is browned on the bottom, stir and continue cooking until it's crisp in parts.
12. Add the sauce from the pot. Serve with the sour cream and diced avocado.

Per Serving
calories: 332 | fat: 23.0g | protein: 26.0g | carbs: 8.0g | net carbs: 5.0g | fiber: 3.0g

Herbed Pork Roast with Asparagus

Prep time: 25 minutes | Cook time: 17 minutes | Serves 6

- 1 teaspoon dried thyme
- ½ teaspoon garlic powder
- ½ teaspoon onion powder
- ½ teaspoon dried oregano
- 1½ teaspoons smoked paprika
- ½ teaspoon ground black pepper
- 1 teaspoon sea salt
- 2 tablespoons olive oil, divided

- 2 pounds (907 g) boneless pork loin roast
- ½ medium white onion, chopped
- 2 garlic cloves, minced
- ⅔ cup chicken broth
- 2 tablespoons Worcestershire sauce
- 1 cup water
- 20 fresh asparagus spears, cut in half and woody ends removed

1. In a small bowl, combine the thyme, garlic powder, onion powder, oregano, smoked paprika, black pepper, and sea salt. Mix until well combined and then add 1½ tablespoons olive oil. Stir until blended.
2. Brush all sides of the pork roast with the oil and spice mixture. Place the roast in a covered dish and transfer to the refrigerator to marinate for 30 minutes.
3. Select Sauté mode and brush the Instant Pot with remaining olive oil. Once the oil is hot, add the pork roast and sear for 5 minutes per side or until browned. Remove the roast from the pot and set aside.
4. Add the onions and garlic to the pot and Sauté for 2 minutes, or until the onions soften and garlic becomes fragrant.
5. Add the chicken broth and Worcestershire sauce.
6. Lock the lid. Select Manual mode and set cooking time for 15 minutes on High pressure.
7. When cooking is complete, allow the pressure release naturally for 10 minutes and then release the remaining pressure.
8. Open the lid. Transfer the roast to a cutting board, cover with aluminum foil, and set aside to rest. Transfer the broth to a measuring cup. Set aside.
9. Place the trivet in the Instant Pot and add the water to the bottom of the pot.
10. Place the asparagus in an ovenproof bowl that will fit in the Instant Pot and place the bowl on top of the trivet.
11. Lock the lid. Select Steam mode and set cooking time for 2 minutes. Once the cook time is complete, quick release the pressure.
12. Open the lid and transfer the asparagus to a large serving platter. Thinly slice the roast and transfer to the serving platter with the asparagus. Drizzle the reserved broth over top. Serve warm.

Per Serving

calories: 257 | fat: 10.8g | protein: 34.6g | carbs: 3.8g | net carbs: 3.0g | fiber: 0.8g

Italian Sausage Stuffed Bell Peppers

Prep time: 15 minutes | Cook time: 17 minutes | Serves 4

- ✿ 4 medium bell peppers, tops and seeds removed
- ✿ 1 pound (454 g) ground pork sausage
- ✿ 1 large egg
- ✿ 3 tablespoons unsweetened tomato purée
- ✿ 2 garlic cloves, minced
- ✿ ½ tablespoon Italian seasoning blend
- ✿ ½ teaspoon sea salt
- ✿ ¼ teaspoon ground black pepper
- ✿ ½ teaspoon onion powder
- ✿ ⅓ cup tomato, puréed
- ✿ 1 cup water
- ✿ 4 slices Mozzarella cheese

1. Using a fork, pierce small holes into the bottoms of the peppers. Set aside.
2. In a large mixing bowl, combine the sausage, egg, tomato purée, garlic, Italian seasoning, sea salt, black pepper, and onion powder. Mix to combine.
3. Stuff each bell pepper with the meat mixture.
4. Place the trivet in the Instant Pot and add the water.
5. Place the stuffed peppers on the trivet. Pour the puréed tomato over.
6. Lock the lid. Select Manual mode and set cooking time for 15 minutes on High Pressure.
7. When cooking is complete, allow the pressure to release naturally for 5 minutes and then release the remaining pressure.
8. Open the lid and top each pepper with 1 slice of the Mozzarella. Secure the lid, select Keep Warm / Cancel, and set cooking time for 2 minutes to melt the cheese.
9. Open the lid and use tongs to carefully transfer the peppers to a large serving platter. Serve warm.

Per Serving
calories: 369 | fat: 22.0g | protein: 17.0g | carbs: 25.8g | net carbs: 8.0g | fiber: 17.8g

Cheesy Pork Taco Casserole

Prep time: 15 minutes | Cook time: 30 minutes | Serves 6

- ✿ ½ cup water
- ✿ 2 eggs
- ✿ 3 ounces (85 g) Cottage cheese, at room temperature
- ✿ ¼ cup heavy cream
- ✿ 1 teaspoon taco seasoning
- ✿ 6 ounces (170 g) Cotija cheese, crumbled
- ✿ ¾ pound (340 g) ground pork
- ✿ ½ cup tomatoes, puréed
- ✿ 1 tablespoon taco seasoning
- ✿ 3 ounces (85 g) chopped green chilies
- ✿ 6 ounces (170 g) Queso Manchego cheese, shredded

1. Add the water in the Instant Pot and place in the trivet.
2. In a mixing bowl, combine the eggs, Cottage cheese, heavy cream, and taco seasoning.
3. Lightly grease a casserole dish. Spread the Cotija cheese over the bottom. Stir in the egg mixture.
4. Lower the casserole dish onto the trivet.
5. Secure the lid. Choose Manual mode and set cooking time for 20 minutes on High Pressure.
6. Once cooking is complete, use a quick pressure release. Carefully remove the lid.
7. In the meantime, heat a skillet over a medium-high heat. Brown the ground pork, crumbling with a fork.
8. Add the tomato purée, taco seasoning, and green chilies. Spread the mixture over the prepared cheese crust.
9. Top with shredded Queso Manchego.
10. Secure the lid. Choose Manual mode and set cooking time for 10 minutes on High Pressure.
11. Once cooking is complete, use a quick pressure release. Carefully remove the lid.
12. Serve immediately.

Per Serving

calories: 409 | fat: 31.6g | protein: 25.7g | carbs: 4.7g | net carbs: 2.7g | fiber: 2.0g

Chile Verde Pulled Pork with Tomatillos

Prep time: 15 minutes | Cook time: 1 hour 3 minutes | Serves 6

- ✿ 2 pounds (907 g) pork shoulder, cut into 6 equal-sized pieces
- ✿ 1 teaspoon sea salt
- ✿ ½ teaspoon ground black pepper
- ✿ 2 jalapeño peppers, deseeded and stemmed
- ✿ 1 pound (454 g) tomatillos, husks removed and quartered
- ✿ 3 garlic cloves
- ✿ 1 tablespoon lime juice
- ✿ 3 tablespoons fresh cilantro, chopped
- ✿ 1 medium white onion, chopped
- ✿ 1 teaspoon ground cumin
- ✿ ½ teaspoon dried oregano
- ✿ 1⅔ cups chicken broth
- ✿ 1½ tablespoons olive oil

1. Season the pork pieces with the salt and pepper. Gently rub the seasonings into the pork cuts. Set aside.
2. Combine the jalapeños, tomatillos, garlic cloves, lime juice, cilantro, onions, cumin, oregano, and chicken broth in the blender. Pulse until well combined. Set aside.
3. Select Sauté mode and add the olive oil to the pot. Once the oil is hot, add the pork cuts and sear for 4 minutes per side or until browned.
4. Pour the jalapeño sauce over the pork and lightly stir to coat well.
5. Lock the lid. Select Manual mode and set cooking time for 55 minutes on High Pressure.
6. When cooking is complete, allow the pressure to release naturally for 10 minutes and then release the remaining pressure.
7. Open the lid. Transfer the pork pieces to a cutting board and use two forks to shred the pork.
8. Transfer the shredded pork back to the pot and stir to combine the pork with the sauce. Transfer to a serving platter. Serve warm.

Per Serving

calories: 381 | fat: 24.8g | protein: 29.3g | carbs: 11.1g | net carbs: 8.3g | fiber: 2.8g

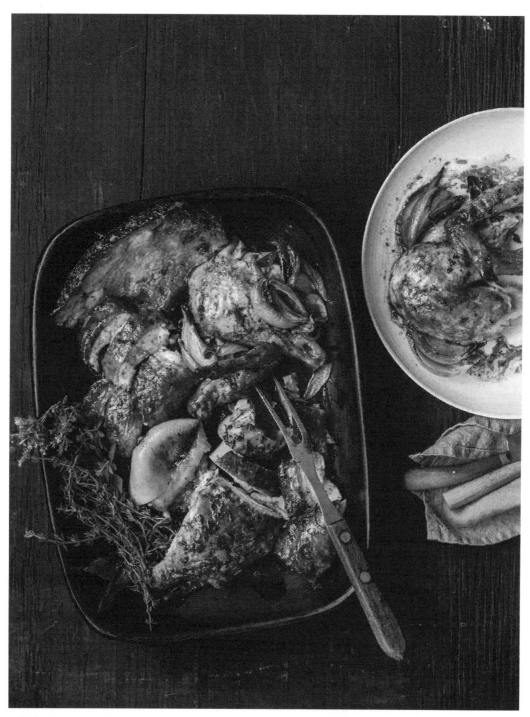

CHAPTER 9
Poultry

Herb and Lemon Whole Chicken

Prep time: 5 minutes | Cook time: 30 to 32 minutes | Serves 4

- 3 teaspoons garlic powder
- 3 teaspoons salt
- 2 teaspoons dried parsley
- 2 teaspoons dried rosemary
- 1 teaspoon pepper
- 1 (4-pound / 1.8-kg) whole chicken
- 2 tablespoons coconut oil
- 1 cup chicken broth
- 1 lemon, zested and quartered

1. Combine the garlic powder, salt, parsley, rosemary, and pepper in a small bowl. Rub this herb mix over the whole chicken.
2. Set your Instant Pot to Sauté and heat the coconut oil.
3. Add the chicken and brown for 5 to 7 minutes. Using tongs, transfer the chicken to a plate.
4. Pour the broth into the Instant Pot and scrape the bottom with a rubber spatula or wooden spoon until no seasoning is stuck to pot, then insert the trivet.
5. Scatter the lemon zest over chicken. Put the lemon quarters inside the chicken. Place the chicken on the trivet.
6. Secure the lid. Select the Meat/Stew mode and set the cooking time for 25 minutes at High Pressure.
7. Once cooking is complete, do a natural pressure release for 10 minutes, then release any remaining pressure. Carefully open the lid.
8. Shred the chicken and serve warm.

Per Serving

calories: 860 | fat: 62.8g | protein: 54.6g | carbs: 3.2g | net carbs: 2.0g | fiber: 1.2g

Barbecue Shredded Chicken

Prep time: 5 minutes | Cook time: 25 minutes | Serves 4

- 1 (5-pound / 2.2-kg) whole chicken
- 3 teaspoons salt
- 1 teaspoon pepper
- 1 teaspoon dried parsley
- 1 teaspoon garlic powder
- ½ medium onion, cut into 3 to 4 large pieces
- 1 cup water
- ½ cup sugar-free barbecue sauce, divided

1. Scatter the chicken with salt, pepper, parsley, and garlic powder. Put the onion pieces inside the chicken cavity.
2. Pour the water into the Instant Pot and insert the trivet. Place seasoned chicken on the trivet. Brush with half of the barbecue sauce.
3. Lock the lid. Select the Manual mode and set the cooking time for 25 minutes at High Pressure.
4. When the timer beeps, perform a natural pressure release for 10 minutes, then release any remaining pressure. Carefully remove the lid.
5. Using a clean brush, add the remaining half of the sauce to chicken. For crispy skin or thicker sauce, you can broil in the oven for 5 minutes until lightly browned.
6. Slice or shred the chicken and serve warm.

Per Serving

calories: 1054 | fat: 73.1g | protein: 70.8g | carbs: 6.6g | net carbs: 5.5g | fiber: 1.1g

Cheesy Chicken Casserole

Prep time: 15 minutes | Cook time: 15 minutes | Serves 4

- ✿ 1 cup broccoli florets
- ✿ 1½ cups Alfredo sauce
- ✿ ½ cup chopped fresh spinach
- ✿ ¼ cup whole-milk ricotta cheese
- ✿ ½ teaspoon salt
- ✿ ¼ teaspoon pepper
- ✿ 1 pound (454 g) thin-sliced deli chicken
- ✿ 1 cup shredded whole-milk Mozzarella cheese
- ✿ 1 cup water

1. Put the broccoli florets in a large bowl. Add the Alfredo sauce, spinach, ricotta, salt, and pepper to the bowl and stir to mix well. Using a spoon, separate the veggie mix into three sections.
2. Layer the chicken into the bottom of a 7-cup glass bowl. Place one section of the veggie mix on top in an even layer and top with a layer of shredded Mozzarella cheese. Repeat until all veggie mix has been used and finish with a layer of Mozzarella cheese. Cover the dish with aluminum foil.
3. Pour the water into the Instant Pot and insert the trivet. Place the dish on the trivet.
4. Secure the lid. Select the Manual mode and set the cooking time for 15 minutes at High Pressure.
5. Once cooking is complete, do a quick pressure release. Carefully open the lid.
6. If desired, broil in oven for 3 to 5 minutes until golden. Serve warm.

Per Serving
calories: 284 | fat: 13.4g | protein: 29.2g | carbs: 9.7g | net carbs: 9.0g | fiber: 0.7g

Chicken Escabèche

Prep time: 5 minutes | Cook time: 15 minutes | Serves 4

- ✿ 1 cup filtered water
- ✿ 1 pound (454 g) chicken, mixed pieces
- ✿ 3 garlic cloves, smashed
- ✿ 2 bay leaves
- ✿ 1 onion, chopped
- ✿ ½ cup red wine vinegar
- ✿ ½ teaspoon coriander
- ✿ ½ teaspoon ground cumin
- ✿ ½ teaspoon mint, finely chopped
- ✿ ½ teaspoon kosher salt
- ✿ ½ teaspoon freshly ground black pepper

1. Pour the water into the Instant Pot and insert the trivet.
2. Thoroughly combine the chicken, garlic, bay leaves, onion, vinegar, coriander, cumin, mint, salt, and black pepper in a large bowl.
3. Put the bowl on the trivet and cover loosely with aluminum foil.
4. Secure the lid. Select the Manual mode and set the cooking time for 15 minutes at High Pressure.
5. Once cooking is complete, do a natural pressure release for 10 minutes, then release any remaining pressure. Carefully open the lid.
6. Remove the dish from the Instant Pot and cool for 5 to 10 minutes before serving.

Per Serving
calories: 196 | fat: 3.7g | protein: 33.5g | carbs: 4.0g | net carbs: 3.3g | fiber: 0.7g

Chicken and Scallions Stuffed Peppers

Prep time: 5 minutes | Cook time: 20 minutes | Serves 5

- 1 tablespoon butter, at room temperature
- ½ cup scallions, chopped
- 1 pound (454 g) ground chicken
- ½ teaspoon sea salt
- ½ teaspoon chili powder
- ⅓ teaspoon paprika
- ⅓ teaspoon ground cumin
- ¼ teaspoon shallot powder
- 6 ounces (170 g) goat cheese, crumbled
- 1½ cups water
- 5 bell peppers, tops, membrane, and seeds removed
- ½ cup sour cream

1. Set your Instant Pot to Sauté and melt the butter.
2. Add the scallions and chicken and sauté for 2 to 3 minutes.
3. Stir in the sea salt, chili powder, paprika, cumin, and shallot powder. Add the crumbled goat cheese, stir, and reserve the mixture in a bowl.
4. Clean your Instant Pot. Pour the water into the Instant Pot and insert the trivet.
5. Stuff the bell peppers with enough of the chicken mixture, and don't pack the peppers too tightly. Put the peppers on the trivet.
6. Lock the lid. Select the Poultry mode and set the cooking time for 15 minutes at High Pressure.
7. When the timer beeps, perform a natural pressure release for 10 minutes, then release any remaining pressure. Carefully remove the lid.
8. Remove from the Instant Pot and serve with the sour cream.

Per Serving
calories: 338 | fat: 19.8g | protein: 30.3g | carbs: 8.6g | net carbs: 7.4g | fiber: 1.2g

Classic Chicken Salad

Prep time: 5 minutes | Cook time: 12 minutes | Serves 8

- 2 pounds (907 g) chicken breasts
- 1 cup vegetable broth
- 2 sprigs fresh thyme
- 1 teaspoon granulated garlic
- 1 teaspoon onion powder
- 1 bay leaf
- ½ teaspoon ground black pepper
- 1 cup mayonnaise
- 2 stalks celery, chopped
- 2 tablespoons chopped fresh chives
- 1 teaspoon fresh lemon juice
- 1 teaspoon Dijon mustard
- ½ teaspoon coarse sea salt

1. Combine the chicken, broth, thyme, garlic, onion powder, bay leaf, and black pepper in the Instant Pot.
2. Lock the lid. Select the Poultry mode and set the cooking time for 12 minutes at High Pressure.
3. When the timer beeps, perform a natural pressure release for 10 minutes, then release any remaining pressure. Carefully remove the lid.
4. Remove the chicken from the Instant Pot and let rest for a few minutes until cooled slightly.
5. Slice the chicken breasts into strips and place in a salad bowl. Add the remaining ingredients and gently stir until well combined. Serve immediately.

Per Serving
calories: 348 | fat: 26.7g | protein: 25.1g | carbs: 1.5g | net carbs: 1.1g | fiber: 0.4g

Spicy Chicken with Bacon and Peppers

Prep time: 5 minutes | Cook time: 13 minutes | Serves 6

- 2 slices bacon, chopped
- 1½ pounds (680 g) ground chicken
- 2 garlic cloves, minced
- ½ cup green onions, chopped
- 1 green bell pepper, seeded and chopped
- 1 red bell pepper, seeded and chopped
- 1 serrano pepper, chopped
- 1 tomato, chopped
- 1 cup water
- ⅓ cup chicken broth
- 1 teaspoon paprika
- 1 teaspoon onion powder
- ¼ teaspoon ground allspice
- 2 bay leaves
- Sea salt and ground black pepper, to taste

1. Press the Sauté button to heat your Instant Pot.
2. Add the bacon and cook for about 3 minutes until crisp. Reserve the bacon in a bowl.
3. Add the ground chicken to the bacon grease of the pot and brown for 2 to 3 minutes, crumbling it with a spatula. Reserve it in the bowl of bacon.
4. Add the garlic, green onions, and peppers and sauté for 3 minutes until tender. Add the remaining ingredients to the Instant Pot, along with the cooked bacon and chicken. Stir to mix well.
5. Lock the lid. Select the Poultry mode and set the cooking time for 5 minutes at High Pressure.
6. When the timer beeps, perform a natural pressure release for 10 minutes, then release any remaining pressure. Carefully remove the lid. Serve warm.

Per Serving

calories: 236 | fat: 13.8g | protein: 24.9g | carbs: 3.0g | net carbs: 2.0g | fiber: 1.0g

Chicken Tacos with Fried Cheese Shells

Prep time: 5 minutes | Cook time: 25 minutes | Serves 6

Chicken:
- 4 (6-ounce / 170-g) boneless, skinless chicken breasts
- 1 cup chicken broth
- 1 teaspoon salt
- ¼ teaspoon pepper
- 1 tablespoon chili powder
- 2 teaspoons garlic powder
- 2 teaspoons cumin

Cheese Shells:
- 1½ cups shredded whole-milk Mozzarella cheese

1. Combine all ingredients for the chicken in the Instant Pot.
2. Secure the lid. Select the Manual mode and set the cooking time for 20 minutes at High Pressure.
3. Once cooking is complete, do a quick pressure release. Carefully open the lid.
4. Shred the chicken and serve in bowls or cheese shells.
5. Make the cheese shells: Heat a nonstick skillet over medium heat.
6. Sprinkle ¼ cup of Mozzarella cheese in the skillet and fry until golden. Flip and turn off the heat. Allow the cheese to get brown. Fill with chicken and fold. The cheese will harden as it cools. Repeat with the remaining cheese and filling.
7. Serve warm.

Per Serving

calories: 233 | fat: 8.2g | protein: 32.4g | carbs: 2.4g | net carbs: 1.7g | fiber: 1.7g

Simple Shredded Chicken

Prep time: 5 minutes | Cook time: 14 minutes | Serves 4

- ½ teaspoon salt
- ½ teaspoon pepper
- ½ teaspoon dried oregano
- ½ teaspoon dried basil
- ½ teaspoon garlic powder
- 2 (6-ounce / 170-g) boneless, skinless chicken breasts
- 1 tablespoon coconut oil
- 1 cup water

1. In a small bowl, combine the salt, pepper, oregano, basil, and garlic powder. Rub this mix over both sides of the chicken.
2. Set your Instant Pot to Sauté and heat the coconut oil until sizzling.
3. Add the chicken and sear for 3 to 4 minutes until golden on both sides.
4. Remove the chicken and set aside.
5. Pour the water into the Instant Pot and use a wooden spoon or rubber spatula to make sure no seasoning is stuck to bottom of pot.
6. Add the trivet to the Instant Pot and place the chicken on top.
7. Secure the lid. Select the Manual mode and set the cooking time for 10 minutes at High Pressure.
8. Once cooking is complete, do a natural pressure release for 5 minutes, then release any remaining pressure. Carefully open the lid.
9. Remove the chicken and shred, then serve.

Per Serving

calories: 135 | fat: 4.8g | protein: 19.7g | carbs: 0.5g | net carbs: 0.3g | fiber: 0.2g

---

Thai Coconut Chicken

Prep time: 10 minutes | Cook time: 15 minutes | Serves 4

- 1 tablespoon coconut oil
- 1 pound (454 g) chicken, cubed
- 2 cloves garlic, minced
- 1 shallot, peeled and chopped
- 1 teaspoon Thai chili, minced
- 1 teaspoon fresh ginger root, julienned
- ⅓ teaspoon cumin powder
- 1 tomato, peeled and chopped
- 1 cup vegetable broth
- ⅓ cup unsweetened coconut milk
- 2 tablespoons coconut aminos
- 1 teaspoon Thai curry paste
- Salt and freshly ground black pepper, to taste

1. Set your Instant Pot to Sauté and heat the coconut oil.
2. Brown the chicken cubes for 2 to 3 minutes, stirring frequently. Reserve the chicken in a bowl.
3. Add the garlic and shallot and sauté for 2 minutes until tender. Add a splash of vegetable broth to the pot, if needed.
4. Stir in the Thai chili, ginger, and cumin powder and cook for another 1 minute or until fragrant.
5. Add the cooked chicken, tomato, vegetable broth, milk, coconut aminos, and curry paste to the Instant Pot and stir well.
6. Lock the lid. Select the Manual mode and set the cooking time for 10 minutes at High Pressure.
7. When the timer beeps, perform a quick pressure release. Carefully remove the lid.
8. Season with salt and pepper to taste and serve.

Per Serving

calories: 196 | fat: 7.7g | protein: 25.9g | carbs: 4.5g | net carbs: 2.9g | fiber: 1.6g

Chicken and Bacon Ranch Casserole

Prep time: 5 minutes | Cook time: 30 minutes | Serves 4

- ✿ 4 slices bacon
- ✿ 4 (6-ounce / 170-g) boneless, skinless chicken breasts, cut into 1-inch cubes
- ✿ ½ teaspoon salt
- ✿ ¼ teaspoon pepper
- ✿ 1 tablespoon coconut oil
- ✿ ½ cup chicken broth
- ✿ ½ cup ranch dressing
- ✿ ½ cup shredded Cheddar cheese
- ✿ 2 ounces (57 g) cream cheese

1. Press the Sauté button to heat your Instant Pot.
2. Add the bacon slices and cook for about 7 minutes until crisp, flipping occasionally.
3. Remove from the pot and place on a paper towel to drain. Set aside.
4. Season the chicken cubes with salt and pepper.
5. Set your Instant Pot to Sauté and melt the coconut oil.
6. Add the chicken cubes and brown for 3 to 4 minutes until golden brown.
7. Stir in the broth and ranch dressing.
8. Secure the lid. Select the Manual mode and set the cooking time for 20 minutes at High Pressure.
9. Once cooking is complete, do a quick pressure release. Carefully open the lid.
10. Stir in the Cheddar and cream cheese. Crumble the cooked bacon and scatter on top. Serve immediately.

Per Serving

calories: 467 | fat: 25.8g | protein: 46.2g | carbs: 1.3g | net carbs: 1.2g | fiber: 0.1g

Keto Chicken Enchilada Bowl

Prep time: 10 minutes | Cook time: 35 minutes | Serves 4

- ✿ 2 (6-ounce / 170-g) boneless, skinless chicken breasts
- ✿ 2 teaspoons chili powder
- ✿ ½ teaspoon garlic powder
- ✿ ½ teaspoon salt
- ✿ ¼ teaspoon pepper
- ✿ 2 tablespoons coconut oil
- ✿ ¾ cup red enchilada sauce
- ✿ ¼ cup chicken broth
- ✿ 1 (4-ounce / 113-g) can green chilies
- ✿ ¼ cup diced onion
- ✿ 2 cups cooked cauliflower rice
- ✿ 1 avocado, diced
- ✿ ½ cup sour cream
- ✿ 1 cup shredded Cheddar cheese

1. Sprinkle the chili powder, garlic powder, salt, and pepper on chicken breasts.
2. Set your Instant Pot to Sauté and melt the coconut oil. Add the chicken breasts and sear each side for about 5 minutes until golden brown.
3. Pour the enchilada sauce and broth over the chicken. Using a wooden spoon or rubber spatula, scrape the bottom of pot to make sure nothing is sticking. Stir in the chilies and onion.
4. Secure the lid. Select the Manual mode and set the cooking time for 25 minutes at High Pressure.
5. Once cooking is complete, do a quick pressure release. Carefully open the lid.
6. Remove the chicken and shred with two forks. Serve the chicken over the cauliflower rice and place the avocado, sour cream, and Cheddar cheese on top.

Per Serving

calories: 434 | fat: 26.1g | protein: 29.3g | carbs: 11.8g | net carbs: 7.0g | fiber: 4.8g

Chicken Piccata

Prep time: 5 minutes | Cook time: 25 minutes | Serves 4

- ✿ 4 (6-ounce / 170-g) boneless, skinless chicken breasts
- ✿ ½ teaspoon salt
- ✿ ½ teaspoon garlic powder
- ✿ ¼ teaspoon pepper
- ✿ 2 tablespoons coconut oil
- ✿ 1 cup water
- ✿ 2 cloves garlic, minced
- ✿ 4 tablespoons butter
- ✿ Juice of 1 lemon
- ✿ ¼ teaspoon xanthan gum

1. Sprinkle the chicken with salt, garlic powder, and pepper.
2. Set your Instant Pot to Sauté and melt the coconut oil.
3. Add the chicken and sear each side for about 5 to 7 minutes until golden brown.
4. Remove the chicken and set aside on a plate.
5. Pour the water into the Instant Pot. Using a wooden spoon, scrape the bottom if necessary to remove any stuck-on seasoning or meat. Insert the trivet and place the chicken on the trivet.
6. Secure the lid. Select the Manual mode and set the cooking time for 10 minutes at High Pressure.
7. Once cooking is complete, do a natural pressure release for 10 minutes, then release any remaining pressure. Carefully open the lid.
8. Remove the chicken and set aside. Strain the broth from the Instant Pot into a large bowl and return to the pot.
9. Set your Instant Pot to Sauté again and add the remaining ingredients. Cook for at least 5 minutes, stirring frequently, or until the sauce is cooked to your desired thickness.
10. Pour the sauce over the chicken and serve warm.

Per Serving

calories: 338 | fat: 19.6g | protein: 32.2g | carbs: 1.8g | net carbs: 1.3g | fiber: 0.5g

Cheesy Pesto Chicken

Prep time: 5 minutes | Cook time: 25 minutes | Serves 2

- 2 (6-ounce / 170-g) boneless, skinless chicken breasts, butterflied
- ½ teaspoon salt
- ¼ teaspoon pepper
- ¼ teaspoon dried parsley
- ¼ teaspoon garlic powder
- 2 tablespoons coconut oil
- 1 cup water
- ¼ cup whole-milk ricotta cheese
- ¼ cup pesto
- ¼ cup shredded whole-milk Mozzarella cheese
- Chopped parsley, for garnish (optional)

1. Sprinkle the chicken breasts with salt, pepper, parsley, and garlic powder.
2. Set your Instant Pot to Sauté and melt the coconut oil.
3. Add the chicken and brown for 3 to 5 minutes. Remove the chicken from the pot to a 7-cup glass bowl.
4. Pour the water into the Instant Pot and use a wooden spoon or rubber spatula to make sure no seasoning is stuck to bottom of pot.
5. Scatter the ricotta cheese on top of the chicken. Pour the pesto over chicken, and sprinkle the Mozzarella cheese over chicken. Cover with aluminum foil. Add the trivet to the Instant Pot and place the bowl on the trivet.
6. Secure the lid. Select the Manual mode and set the cooking time for 20 minutes at High Pressure.
7. Once cooking is complete, do a natural pressure release for 10 minutes, then release any remaining pressure. Carefully open the lid.
8. Serve the chicken garnished with the chopped parsley, if desired.

Per Serving
calories: 519 | fat: 31.9g | protein: 46.4g | carbs: 4.2g | net carbs: 3.5g | fiber: 0.7g

Chicken Alfredo with Bacon

Prep time: 10 minutes | Cook time: 27 minutes | Serves 4

- ✿ 2 (6-ounce / 170-g) boneless, skinless chicken breasts, butterflied
- ✿ ½ teaspoon garlic powder
- ✿ ¼ teaspoon dried parsley
- ✿ ¼ teaspoon dried thyme
- ✿ ¼ teaspoon salt
- ✿ ⅛ teaspoon pepper
- ✿ 2 tablespoons coconut oil
- ✿ 1 cup water
- ✿ 1 stick butter
- ✿ 2 cloves garlic, finely minced
- ✿ ¼ cup heavy cream
- ✿ ½ cup grated Parmesan cheese
- ✿ ¼ cup cooked crumbled bacon

1. Sprinkle the chicken breasts with the garlic powder, parsley, thyme, salt, and pepper.
2. Set your Instant Pot to Sauté and melt the coconut oil.
3. Add the chicken and sear for 3 to 5 minutes until golden brown on both sides.
4. Remove the chicken with tongs and set aside.
5. Pour the water into the Instant Pot and insert the trivet. Place the chicken on the trivet.
6. Secure the lid. Select the Manual mode and set the cooking time for 20 minutes at High Pressure.
7. Once cooking is complete, do a quick pressure release. Carefully open the lid.
8. Remove the chicken from the pot to a platter and set aside.
9. Pour the water out of the Instant Pot, reserving ½ cup; set aside.
10. Set your Instant Pot to Sauté again and melt the butter.
11. Add the garlic, heavy cream, cheese, and reserved water to the Instant Pot. Cook for 3 to 4 minutes until the sauce starts to thicken, stirring frequently.
12. Stir in the crumbled bacon and pour the mixture over the chicken. Serve immediately.

Per Serving

calories: 526| fat: 41.6g | protein: 27.7g | carbs: 3.0g | net carbs: 2.9g | fiber: 0.1g

Stuffed Chicken with Spinach and Feta

Prep time: 10 minutes | Cook time: 25 minutes | Serves 4

- ✿ ½ cup frozen spinach
- ✿ ⅓ cup crumbled feta cheese
- ✿ 1¼ teaspoons salt, divided
- ✿ 4 (6-ounce / 170-g) boneless, skinless chicken breasts, butterflied
- ✿ ¼ teaspoon pepper
- ✿ ¼ teaspoon dried oregano
- ✿ ¼ teaspoon dried parsley
- ✿ ¼ teaspoon garlic powder
- ✿ 2 tablespoons coconut oil
- ✿ 1 cup water

1. Combine the spinach, feta cheese, and ¼ teaspoon of salt in a medium bowl. Divide the mixture evenly and spoon onto the chicken breasts.
2. Close the chicken breasts and secure with toothpicks or butcher's string. Sprinkle the chicken with the remaining 1 teaspoon of salt, pepper, oregano, parsley, and garlic powder.
3. Set your Instant Pot to Sauté and heat the coconut oil.
4. Sear each chicken breast until golden brown, about 4 to 5 minutes per side.
5. Remove the chicken breasts and set aside.
6. Pour the water into the Instant Pot and scrape the bottom to remove any chicken or seasoning that is stuck on. Add the trivet to the Instant Pot and place the chicken on the trivet.
7. Secure the lid. Select the Manual mode and set the cooking time for 15 minutes at High Pressure.
8. Once cooking is complete, do a natural pressure release for 15 minutes, then release any remaining pressure. Carefully open the lid. Serve warm.

Per Serving

calories: 303 | fat: 12.1g | protein: 40.9g | carbs: 1.3g | net carbs: 0.6g | fiber: 0.7g

BLT Chicken Salad

Prep time: 15 minutes | Cook time: 17 minutes | Serves 4

- ✿ 4 slices bacon
- ✿ 2 (6-ounce / 170-g) chicken breasts
- ✿ 1 teaspoon salt
- ✿ ½ teaspoon garlic powder
- ✿ ¼ teaspoon dried parsley
- ✿ ¼ teaspoon pepper
- ✿ ¼ teaspoon dried thyme
- ✿ 1 cup water
- ✿ 2 cups chopped romaine lettuce

Sauce:
- ✿ ⅓ cup mayonnaise
- ✿ 1 ounce (28 g) chopped pecans
- ✿ ½ cup diced Roma tomatoes
- ✿ ½ avocado, diced
- ✿ 1 tablespoon lemon juice

1. Press the Sauté button to heat your Instant Pot.
2. Add the bacon and cook for about 7 minutes, flipping occasionally, until crisp. Remove and place on a paper towel to drain. When cool enough to handle, crumble the bacon and set aside.
3. Sprinkle the chicken with salt, garlic powder, parsley, pepper, and thyme.
4. Pour the water into the Instant Pot. Use a wooden spoon to ensure nothing is stuck to the bottom of the pot. Add the trivet to the pot and place the chicken on top of the trivet.
5. Secure the lid. Select the Manual mode and set the cooking time for 10 minutes at High Pressure.
6. Meanwhile, whisk together all the ingredients for the sauce in a large salad bowl.
7. Once cooking is complete, do a quick pressure release. Carefully open the lid.
8. Remove the chicken and let sit for 10 minutes. Cut the chicken into cubes and transfer to the salad bowl, along with the cooked bacon. Gently stir until the chicken is thoroughly coated. Mix in the lettuce right before serving.

Per Serving
calories: 431 | fat: 32.6g | protein: 24.3g | carbs: 5.1g | net carbs: 2.4g | fiber: 2.7g

Baked Cheesy Mushroom Chicken

Prep time: 5 minutes | Cook time: 15 minutes | Serves 4

- ✿ 1 tablespoon butter
- ✿ 2 cloves garlic, smashed
- ✿ ½ cup chopped yellow onion
- ✿ 1 pound (454 g) chicken breasts, cubed
- ✿ 10 ounces (283 g) button mushrooms, thinly sliced
- ✿ 1 cup chicken broth
- ✿ ½ teaspoon shallot powder
- ✿ ½ teaspoon turmeric powder
- ✿ ½ teaspoon dried basil
- ✿ ½ teaspoon dried sage
- ✿ ½ teaspoon cayenne pepper
- ✿ ⅓ teaspoon ground black pepper
- ✿ Kosher salt, to taste
- ✿ ½ cup heavy cream
- ✿ 1 cup shredded Colby cheese

1. Set your Instant Pot to Sauté and melt the butter.
2. Add the garlic, onion, chicken, and mushrooms and sauté for about 4 minutes, or until the vegetables are softened.
3. Add the remaining ingredients except the heavy cream and cheese to the Instant Pot and stir to incorporate.
4. Lock the lid. Select the Meat/Stew mode and set the cooking time for 6 minutes at High Pressure.
5. When the timer beeps, perform a natural pressure release for 10 minutes, then release any remaining pressure. Carefully remove the lid.
6. Stir in the heavy cream until heated through. Pour the mixture into a baking dish and scatter the cheese on top.
7. Bake in the preheated oven at 400ºF (205ºC) until the cheese bubbles.
8. Allow to cool for 5 minutes and serve.

Per Serving
calories: 439 | fat: 28.8g | protein: 34.5g | carbs: 10.5g | net carbs: 8.4g | fiber: 2.1g

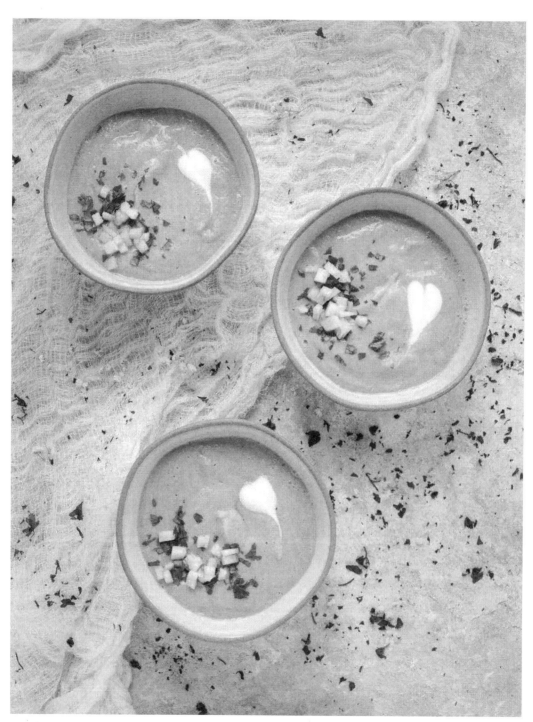

CHAPTER 10
Soups and Stews

Avocado and Serrano Chile Soup

Prep time: 10 minutes | Cook time: 7 minutes | Serves 4

- 2 avocados
- 1 small fresh tomatillo, quartered
- 2 cups chicken broth
- 2 tablespoons avocado oil
- 1 tablespoon butter
- 2 tablespoons finely minced onion
- 1 clove garlic, minced
- ½ Serrano chile, deseeded and ribs removed, minced, plus thin slices for garnish
- ¼ teaspoon sea salt
- Pinch of ground white pepper
- ½ cup full-fat coconut milk
- Fresh cilantro sprigs, for garnish

1. Scoop the avocado flesh into a food processor. Add the tomatillo and chicken broth and purée until smooth. Set aside.
2. Set the Instant Pot to Sauté mode and add the avocado oil and butter. When the butter melts, add the onion and garlic and sauté for a minute or until softened. Add the Serrano chile and sauté for 1 minute more.
3. Pour the puréed avocado mixture into the pot, add the salt and pepper, and stir to combine.
4. Secure the lid. Press the Manual button and set cooking time for 5 minutes on High Pressure.
5. When timer beeps, use a quick pressure release. Open the lid and stir in the coconut milk.
6. Serve hot topped with thin slices of Serrano chile, and cilantro sprigs.

Per Serving

calories: 333 | fat: 32.1g | protein: 3.8g | carbs: 14.5g | net carbs: 6.6g | fiber: 7.9g

Leek and Jack Cheese Soup

Prep time: 10 minutes | Cook time: 15 minutes | Serves 4

- 4 tablespoons butter
- 7 ounces (198 g) leek, chopped
- ½ teaspoon salt
- 1 teaspoon Italian seasonings
- 2 cups chicken broth
- 2 ounces (57 g) Monterey Jack cheese, shredded

1. Heat the butter in the Instant Pot for 4 minutes or until melted.
2. Add the chopped leek, salt, and Italian seasonings.
3. Sauté the leek on Sauté mode for 5 minutes.
4. Pour in the chicken broth and close the lid.
5. Select Manual mode and set cooking time for 10 minutes on High Pressure.
6. When timer beeps, use a quick pressure release. Open the lid.
7. Add the shredded cheese and stir until the cheese is melted.
8. Serve immediately.

Per Serving

calories: 208 | fat: 17.0g | protein: 6.8g | carbs: 7.7g | net carbs: 6.8g | fiber: 0.9g

Bacon, Leek, and Cauliflower Soup

Prep time: 15 minutes | Cook time: 15 minutes | Serves 6

- 6 slices bacon
- 1 leek, remove the dark green end and roots, sliced in half lengthwise, rinsed, cut into ½-inch-thick slices crosswise
- ½ medium yellow onion, sliced
- 4 cloves garlic, minced
- 3 cups chicken broth
- 1 large head cauliflower, roughly chopped into florets
- 1 cup water
- 1 teaspoon kosher salt
- 1 teaspoon ground black pepper
- ⅔ cup shredded sharp Cheddar cheese, divided
- ½ cup heavy whipping cream

1. Set the Instant Pot to Sauté mode. When heated, place the bacon on the bottom of the pot and cook for 5 minutes or until crispy.
2. Transfer the bacon slices to a plate. Let stand until cool enough to handle, crumble it with forks.
3. Add the leek and onion to the bacon fat remaining in the pot. Sauté for 5 minutes or until fragrant and the onion begins to caramelize. Add the garlic and sauté for 30 seconds more or until fragrant.
4. Stir in the chicken broth, cauliflower florets, water, salt, pepper, and three-quarters of the crumbled bacon.
5. Secure the lid. Press the Manual button and set cooking time for 3 minutes on High Pressure.
6. When timer beeps, perform a quick pressure release. Open the lid.
7. Stir in ½ cup of the Cheddar and the cream. Use an immersion blender to purée the soup until smooth.
8. Ladle into bowls and garnish with the remaining Cheddar and crumbled bacon. Serve immediately.

Per Serving
calories: 251 | fat: 18.9g | protein: 10.5g | carbs: 12.0g | net carbs: 8.6g | fiber: 3.4g

Beef and Okra Stew

Prep time: 15 minutes | Cook time: 25 minutes | Serves 3

- 8 ounces (227 g) beef sirloin, chopped
- ¼ teaspoon cumin seeds
- 1 teaspoon dried basil
- 1 tablespoon avocado oil
- ¼ cup coconut cream
- 1 cup water
- 6 ounces (170 g) okra, chopped

1. Sprinkle the beef sirloin with cumin seeds and dried basil and put in the Instant Pot.
2. Add avocado oil and roast the meat on Sauté mode for 5 minutes. Flip occasionally.
3. Add coconut cream, water, and okra.
4. Close the lid and select Manual mode. Set cooking time for 25 minutes on High Pressure.
5. When timer beeps, use a natural pressure release for 10 minutes, the release any remaining pressure. Open the lid.
6. Serve warm.

Per Serving
calories: 216 | fat: 10.2g | protein: 24.6g | carbs: 5.7g | net carbs: 3.2g | fiber: 2.5g

Blue Cheese Mushroom Soup

Prep time: 15 minutes | Cook time: 20 minutes | Serves 4

- ✿ 2 cups chopped white mushrooms
- ✿ 3 tablespoons cream cheese
- ✿ 4 ounces (113 g) scallions, diced
- ✿ 4 cups chicken broth
- ✿ 1 teaspoon olive oil
- ✿ ½ teaspoon ground cumin
- ✿ 1 teaspoon salt
- ✿ 2 ounces (57 g) blue cheese, crumbled

1. Combine the mushrooms, cream cheese, scallions, chicken broth, olive oil, and ground cumin in the Instant Pot.
2. Seal the lid. Select Manual mode and set cooking time for 20 minutes on High Pressure.
3. When timer beeps, use a quick pressure release and open the lid.
4. Add the salt and blend the soup with an immersion blender.
5. Ladle the soup in the bowls and top with blue cheese. Serve warm.

Per Serving

calories: 142 | fat: 9.4g | protein: 10.1g | carbs: 4.8g | net carbs: 3.7g | fiber: 1.1g

---

Broccoli and Bacon Cheese Soup

Prep time: 6 minutes | Cook time: 10 minutes | Serves 6

- ✿ 3 tablespoons butter
- ✿ 2 stalks celery, diced
- ✿ ½ yellow onion, diced
- ✿ 3 garlic cloves, minced
- ✿ 3½ cups chicken stock
- ✿ 4 cups chopped fresh broccoli florets
- ✿ 3 ounces (85 g) block-style cream cheese, softened and cubed
- ✿ ½ teaspoon ground nutmeg
- ✿ ½ teaspoon sea salt
- ✿ 1 teaspoon ground black pepper
- ✿ 3 cups shredded Cheddar cheese
- ✿ ½ cup shredded Monterey Jack cheese
- ✿ 2 cups heavy cream
- ✿ 4 slices cooked bacon, crumbled
- ✿ 1 tablespoon finely chopped chives

1. Select Sauté mode. Once the Instant Pot is hot, add the butter and heat until the butter is melted.
2. Add the celery, onions, and garlic. Continue sautéing for 5 minutes or until the vegetables are softened.
3. Add the chicken stock and broccoli florets to the pot. Bring the liquid to a boil.
4. Lock the lid,. Select Manual mode and set cooking time for 5 minutes on High Pressure.
5. When cooking is complete, allow the pressure to release naturally for 10 minutes and then release the remaining pressure.
6. Open the lid and add the cream cheese, nutmeg, sea salt, and black pepper. Stir to combine.
7. Select Sauté mode. Bring the soup to a boil and then slowly stir in the Cheddar and Jack cheeses. Once the cheese has melted, stir in the heavy cream.
8. Ladle the soup into serving bowls and top with bacon and chives. Serve hot.

Per Serving

calories: 681 | fat: 59.0g | protein: 27.4g | carbs: 11.6g | net carbs: 10.3g | fiber: 1.3g

Cauliflower Rice and Chicken Thigh Soup

Prep time: 15 minutes | Cook time: 13 minutes | Serves 5

- 2 cups cauliflower florets
- 1 pound (454 g) boneless, skinless chicken thighs
- 4½ cups chicken broth
- ½ yellow onion, chopped
- 2 garlic cloves, minced
- 1 tablespoon unflavored gelatin powder
- 2 teaspoons sea salt
- ½ teaspoon ground black pepper
- ½ cup sliced zucchini
- ⅓ cup sliced turnips
- 1 teaspoon dried parsley
- 3 celery stalks, chopped
- 1 teaspoon ground turmeric
- ½ teaspoon dried marjoram
- 1 teaspoon dried thyme
- ½ teaspoon dried oregano

1. Add the cauliflower florets to a food processor and pulse until a ricelike consistency is achieved. Set aside.
2. Add the chicken thighs, chicken broth, onions, garlic, gelatin powder, sea salt, and black pepper to the pot. Gently stir to combine.
3. Lock the lid. Select Manual mode and set cooking time for 10 minutes on High Pressure.
4. When cooking is complete, quick release the pressure and open the lid.
5. Transfer the chicken thighs to a cutting board. Chop the chicken into bite-sized pieces and then return the chopped chicken to the pot.
6. Add the cauliflower rice, zucchini, turnips, parsley, celery, turmeric, marjoram, thyme, and oregano to the pot. Stir to combine.
7. Lock the lid. Select Manual mode and set cooking time for 3 minutes on High Pressure.
8. When cooking is complete, quick release the pressure.
9. Open the lid. Ladle the soup into serving bowls. Serve hot.

Per Serving

calories: 247 | fat: 10.4g | protein: 30.2g | carbs: 8.3g | net carbs: 6.1g | fiber: 2.2g

Chicken Chili Verde Soup

Prep time: 10 minutes | Cook time: 25 minutes | Serves 4

- 1 pound (454 g) chicken breast, skinless, boneless
- 5 cups chicken broth
- ½ cup Cheddar cheese, shredded
- 2 ounces (57 g) chili Verde sauce
- 1 tablespoon dried cilantro

1. Put chicken breast and chicken broth in the Instant Pot.
2. Add the cilantro, Close the lid. Select Manual mode and set cooking time for 15 minutes on High Pressure.
3. When timer beeps, make a quick pressure release and open the lid.
4. Shred the chicken breast with a fork.
5. Add the Cheddar and chili Verde sauce in the soup and cook on Sauté mode for 10 minutes.
6. Mix in the dried cilantro. Serve immediately.

Per Serving

calories: 257 | fat: 10.2g | protein: 34.5g | carbs: 4.0g | net carbs: 3.8g | fiber: 0.2g

Creamy Bacon and Cauliflower Chowder

Prep time: 10 minutes | Cook time: 25 minutes | Serves 6

- 2 cups chicken broth
- 8 ounces (227 g) diced bacon, uncooked
- 5 ounces (142 g) diced onion (about 1 small onion)
- 1 teaspoon salt
- ½ teaspoon black pepper
- 1 (2-pound / 907-g) large head cauliflower, stem and core removed, cut into florets
- 8 ounces (227 g) cream cheese, softened and cut into small cubes
- ½ cup heavy cream, at room temperature

1. Pour the chicken broth into the pot. Add the bacon, onion, salt, and pepper. Stir to combine. Place the large florets in the pot.
2. Close the lid. Select Manual mode and set cooking time for 25 minutes on High Pressure.
3. When timer beeps, perform a quick pressure release. Open the lid.
4. Use a potato masher to break the cauliflower apart into little pieces.
5. Stir in the cream cheese and heavy cream. Serve warm.

Per Serving

calories: 328 | fat: 24.6g | protein: 16.3g | carbs: 9.1g | net carbs: 6.4g | fiber: 2.7g

---

Hearty Chuck Roast and Vegetable Stew

Prep time: 20 minutes | Cook time: 40 minutes | Serves 4

- 1 pound (454 g) beef chuck roast, cut into 1-inch cubes
- 2 teaspoons arrowroot powder
- 1½ tablespoons olive oil
- 1 cup chopped mushrooms
- 1 cup chopped zucchini
- ½ cup sliced turnips
- 3 ribs celery, sliced
- ¾ cup unsweetened tomato purée
- 4 cups beef broth
- 2 garlic cloves, minced
- 1 tablespoon dried thyme
- 1 tablespoon paprika
- 1 teaspoon dried rosemary
- 1 teaspoon dried parsley
- 1 teaspoon garlic powder
- 1 teaspoon celery seed
- 1 teaspoon onion powder
- 2½ teaspoons sea salt
- 1 teaspoon ground black pepper

1. In a large bowl, combine the chuck roast and arrowroot powder. Toss to coat well.
2. Select Sauté mode and add the olive oil to the pot. Once the oil is hot, add the meat and sauté for 5 minutes or until the meat is browned on all sides.
3. Once the meat is browned, add the mushrooms, zucchini, turnips, celery, tomato purée, beef broth, garlic, thyme, paprika, rosemary, parsley, garlic powder, celery seed, sea salt, black pepper, and onion powder to the pot. Stir well to combine.
4. Lock the lid. Select Meat/Stew and set cooking time for 35 minutes on High Pressure.
5. When cooking is complete, allow the pressure to release naturally for 15 minutes and then release the remaining pressure.
6. Open the lid, stir, and then ladle the stew into serving bowls. Serve hot.

Per Serving

calories: 313 | fat: 15.9g | protein: 35.6g | carbs: 8.9g | net carbs: 6.2g | fiber: 2.7g

Creamy Beef Soup

Prep time: 15 minutes | Cook time: 20 minutes | Serves 6

- ✿ 1 tablespoon coconut oil
- ✿ 1 cup ground beef
- ✿ 1 teaspoon taco seasonings
- ✿ ½ cup crushed tomatoes

- ✿ 2 tablespoons cream cheese
- ✿ 1 bell pepper, chopped
- ✿ 1 garlic clove, diced
- ✿ 4 cups beef broth

1. Heat the the coconut oil in the Instant Pot on Sauté mode.
2. Add the ground beef and sprinkle with taco seasonings. Stir well and cook the meat on Sauté mode for 5 minutes.
3. Add crushed tomatoes, cream cheese, bell pepper, garlic clove, and beef broth.
4. Close the lid and select Manual mode. Set cooking time for 15 minutes on High Pressure.
5. When cooking is complete, perform a natural pressure release for 10 minutes and open the lid.
6. Ladle the soup and serve.

Per Serving
calories: 117 | fat: 7.1g | protein: 8.6g | carbs: 4.4g | net carbs: 3.4g | fiber: 1.0g

Mexican Chicken and Avocado Soup

Prep time: 15 minutes | Cook time: 25 minutes | Serves 5

- ✿ 2 tablespoons olive oil
- ✿ 1 pound (454 g) boneless, skinless chicken thighs, cut into bite-sized pieces
- ✿ 4 garlic cloves, minced
- ✿ ½ medium yellow onion, diced
- ✿ 2 jalapeño, stems and seeds removed, chopped
- ✿ ½ cup diced fresh tomato

- ✿ 5 cups chicken broth
- ✿ Juice of 2 limes
- ✿ 2 teaspoons sea salt
- ✿ 1 teaspoon chili powder
- ✿ ½ teaspoon garlic powder
- ✿ ¼ teaspoon ground black pepper
- ✿ 1 medium avocado, chopped
- ✿ ⅓ cup shredded pepper Jack cheese

1. Select the Instant Pot on Sauté mode and add the olive oil. Once the oil is hot, add the chicken and sauté for 3 minutes per side or until browned.
2. Add the garlic, onions, and jalapeños to the pot. Continue sautéing or until the vegetables are softened.
3. Add the diced tomatoes, chicken broth, lime juice, sea salt, chili powder, garlic powder, and black pepper. Stir to combine.
4. Lock the lid. Select Manual mode and set cooking time for 20 minutes on High Pressure.
5. When cooking is complete, allow the pressure to release naturally for 15 minutes and then release the remaining pressure.
6. Open the lid and ladle the soup into serving bowls. Top each serving with equal amounts of the avocado and pepper Jack cheese. Serve hot.

Per Serving
calories: 337 | fat: 16.8g | protein: 13.6g | carbs: 28.5g | net carbs: 23.5g | fiber: 5.0g

Green Garden Soup

Prep time: 20 minutes | Cook time: 29 minutes | Serves 5

- ✿ 1 tablespoon olive oil
- ✿ 1 garlic clove, diced
- ✿ ½ cup cauliflower florets
- ✿ 1 cup kale, chopped
- ✿ 2 tablespoons chives, chopped
- ✿ 1 teaspoon sea salt
- ✿ 6 cups beef broth

1. Heat the olive oil in the Instant Pot on Sauté mode for 2 minutes and add the garlic. Sauté for 2 minutes or until fragrant.
2. Add cauliflower, kale, chives, sea salt, and beef broth.
3. Close the lid. Select Manual mode and set cooking time for 5 minutes on High Pressure.
4. When timer beeps, use a quick pressure release and open the lid.
5. Ladle the soup into the bowls. Serve warm.

Per Serving

calories: 80 | fat: 4.5g | protein: 6.5g | carbs: 2.3g | net carbs: 1.8g | fiber: 0.5g

Bacon Curry Soup

Prep time: 10 minutes | Cook time: 20 minutes | Serves 4

- ✿ 3 ounces (85 g) bacon, chopped
- ✿ 1 tablespoon chopped scallions
- ✿ 1 teaspoon curry powder
- ✿ 1 cup coconut milk
- ✿ 3 cups beef broth
- ✿ 1 cup Cheddar cheese, shredded

1. Heat the the Instant Pot on Sauté mode for 3 minutes and add bacon. Cook for 5 minutes. Flip constantly.
2. Add the scallions and curry powder. Sauté for 5 minutes more.
3. Pour in the coconut milk and beef broth. Add the Cheddar cheese and stir to mix well.
4. Select Manual mode and set cooking time for 10 minutes on High Pressure.
5. When timer beeps, use a quick pressure release. Open the lid.
6. Blend the soup with an immersion blender until smooth. Serve warm.

Per Serving

calories: 398 | fat: 33.6g | protein: 20.0g | carbs: 5.1g | net carbs: 3.6g | fiber: 1.5g

Mushroom, Artichoke, and Spinach Soup

Prep time: 15 minutes | Cook time: 20 minutes | Serves 4

- ✿ 3 tablespoons salted butter
- ✿ 8 ounces (227 g) cremini mushrooms, sliced
- ✿ 1 (6-ounce / 170-g) small jar artichoke hearts packed in water or olive oil, drained, chopped
- ✿ 4 ounces (113 g) full-fat cream cheese
- ✿ 1 teaspoon dried sage
- ✿ 1 teaspoon dried thyme
- ✿ 1 tablespoon Dijon mustard
- ✿ ½ teaspoon garlic powder
- ✿ ½ teaspoon kosher salt
- ✿ ¼ teaspoon ground black pepper
- ✿ 2 cups chicken broth
- ✿ 1 cup water
- ✿ 2 cups roughly chopped baby spinach
- ✿ ½ cup heavy whipping cream
- ✿ ½ cup grated Parmesan cheese

1. Set the Instant Pot to Sauté mode and add the butter. When butter melts, add the mushrooms and sauté for about 8 minutes or until soft.
2. Add the cream cheese to the pot and stir until it is melted. Stir in the sage, thyme, mustard, garlic powder, salt, and black pepper, then mix in the bone broth, water, and artichoke hearts.
3. Secure the lid. Press the Manual button and set cooking time for 5 minutes on High Pressure.
4. When timer beeps, allow the pressure to release naturally for 5 minutes, then release any remaining pressure. Open the lid.
5. Stir in the baby spinach and secure the lid. Allow the spinach to cook for 2 minutes in the soup on Keep Warm / Cancel. Open the lid and stir.
6. Use an immersion blender to blend the soup until smooth and creamy. Stir in the cream.
7. To serve, ladle the soup into bowls and sprinkle with Parmesan cheese. Serve hot.

Per Serving

calories: 261 | fat: 19.7g | protein: 10.5g | carbs: 13.2g | net carbs: 9.8g | fiber: 3.4g

Beef Meatball Minestrone

Prep time: 5 minutes | Cook time: 35 minutes | Serves 6

- 1 pound (454 g) ground beef
- 1 large egg
- 1½ tablespoons golden flaxseed meal
- ⅓ cup shredded Mozzarella cheese
- ¼ cup unsweetened tomato purée
- 1½ tablespoons Italian seasoning, divided
- 1½ teaspoons garlic powder, divided
- 1½ teaspoons sea salt, divided
- 1 tablespoon olive oil
- 2 garlic cloves, minced
- ½ medium yellow onion, minced
- ¼ cup pancetta, diced
- 1 cup sliced yellow squash
- 1 cup sliced zucchini
- ½ cup sliced turnips
- 4 cups beef broth
- 14 ounces (397 g) can diced tomatoes
- ½ teaspoon ground black pepper
- 3 tablespoons shredded Parmesan cheese

1. Preheat the oven to 400°F (205°C) and line a large baking sheet with aluminum foil.
2. In a large bowl, combine the ground beef, egg, flaxseed meal, Mozzarella, unsweetened tomato purée, ½ tablespoon of Italian seasoning, ½ teaspoon of garlic powder, and ½ teaspoon of sea salt. Mix the ingredients until well combined.
3. Make the meatballs by shaping 1 heaping tablespoon of the ground beef mixture into a meatball. Repeat with the remaining mixture and then transfer the meatballs to the prepared baking sheet.
4. Place the meatballs in the oven and bake for 15 minutes. When the baking time is complete, remove from the oven and set aside.
5. Select Sauté mode of the Instant Pot. Once the pot is hot, add the olive oil, garlic, onion, and pancetta. Sauté for 2 minutes or until the garlic becomes fragrant and the onions begin to soften.
6. Add the yellow squash, zucchini, and turnips to the pot. Sauté for 3 more minutes.
7. Add the beef broth, diced tomatoes, black pepper, and remaining garlic powder, sea salt, and Italian seasoning to the pot. Stir to combine and then add the meatballs.
8. Lock the lid. Select Manual mode and set cooking time for 15 minutes on High Pressure.
9. When cooking is complete, allow the pressure to release naturally for 10 minutes and then release the remaining pressure.
10. Open the lid and gently stir the soup. Ladle into serving bowls and top with Parmesan. Serve hot.

Per Serving
calories: 373 | fat: 18.8g | protein: 34.7g | carbs: 15.0g | net carbs: 11.3g | fiber: 3.7g

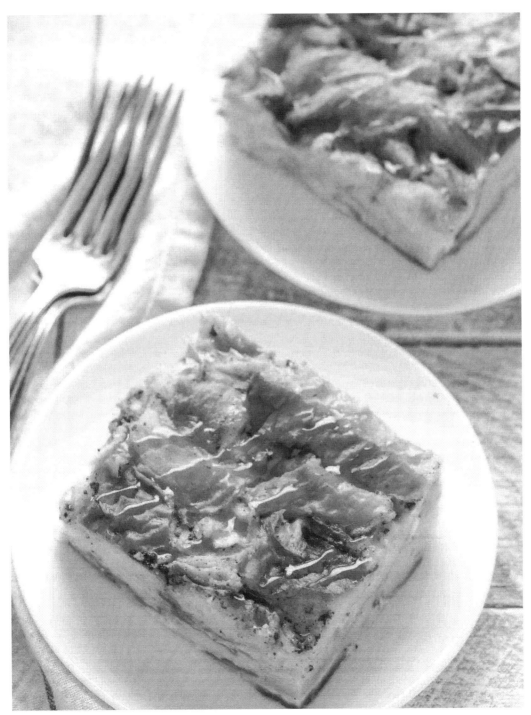

Desserts

Cocoa Custard

Prep time: 5 minutes | Cook time: 7 minutes | Serves 4

- 2 cups heavy cream (or full-fat coconut milk for dairy-free)
- 4 large egg yolks
- ¼ cup Swerve, or more to taste
- 1 tablespoon plus 1 teaspoon unsweetened cocoa powder, or more to taste
- ½ teaspoon almond extract
- Pinch of fine sea salt
- 1 cup cold water

1. Heat the cream in a pan over medium-high heat until hot, about 2 minutes.
2. Place the remaining ingredients except the water in a blender and blend until smooth.
3. While the blender is running, slowly pour in the hot cream. Taste and adjust the sweetness to your liking. Add more cocoa powder, if desired.
4. Scoop the custard mixture into four ramekins with a spatula. Cover the ramekins with aluminum foil.
5. Place a trivet in the Instant Pot and pour in the water. Place the ramekins on the trivet.
6. Lock the lid. Select the Manual mode and set the cooking time for 5 minutes at High Pressure.
7. When the timer beeps, use a quick pressure release. Carefully remove the lid.
8. Remove the foil and set the foil aside. Let the custard cool for 15 minutes. Cover the ramekins with the foil again and place in the refrigerator to chill completely, about 2 hours.
9. Serve.

Per Serving
calories: 269 | fat: 26.9g | protein: 4.1g | carbs: 3.8g | net carbs: 3.6g | fiber: 0.2g

Pumpkin Pie Spice Pots De Crème

Prep time: 5 minutes | Cook time: 7 minutes | Serves 4

- 2 cups heavy cream (or full-fat coconut milk for dairy-free)
- 4 large egg yolks
- ¼ cup Swerve, or more to taste
- 2 teaspoons pumpkin pie spice
- 1 teaspoon vanilla or maple extract
- Pinch of fine sea salt
- 1 cup cold water

1. Heat the cream in a pan over medium-high heat until hot, about 2 minutes.
2. Place the remaining ingredients except the water in a medium bowl and stir until smooth.
3. Slowly pour in the hot cream while stirring. Taste and adjust the sweetness to your liking. Scoop the mixture into four ramekins with a spatula. Cover the ramekins with aluminum foil.
4. Place a trivet in the Instant Pot and pour in the water. Place the ramekins on the trivet.
5. Lock the lid. Select the Manual mode and set the cooking time for 5 minutes at High Pressure.
6. When the timer beeps, use a quick pressure release. Carefully remove the lid.
7. Remove the foil and set the foil aside. Let the pots de crème cool for 15 minutes. Cover the ramekins with the foil again and place in the refrigerator to chill completely, about 2 hours.
8. Serve.

Per Serving
calories: 289 | fat: 27.1g | protein: 7.6g | carbs: 4.0g | net carbs: 3.9g | fiber: 0.1g

Vanilla Crème Brûlée

Prep time: 7 minutes | Cook time: 9 minutes | Serves 4

- ✿ 1 cup heavy cream (or full-fat coconut milk for dairy-free)
- ✿ 2 large egg yolks
- ✿ 2 tablespoons Swerve, or more to taste
- ✿ Seeds scraped from ½ vanilla bean (about 8 inches long), or 1 teaspoon vanilla extract
- ✿ 1 cup cold water
- ✿ 4 teaspoons Swerve, for topping

1. Heat the cream in a pan over medium-high heat until hot, about 2 minutes.
2. Place the egg yolks, Swerve, and vanilla seeds in a blender and blend until smooth.
3. While the blender is running, slowly pour in the hot cream. Taste and adjust the sweetness to your liking.
4. Scoop the mixture into four ramekins with a spatula. Cover the ramekins with aluminum foil.
5. Add the water to the Instant Pot and insert a trivet. Place the ramekins on the trivet.
6. Lock the lid. Select the Manual mode and set the cooking time for 7 minutes at High Pressure.
7. When the timer beeps, perform a quick pressure release. Carefully remove the lid.
8. Keep the ramekins covered with the foil and place in the refrigerator for about 2 hours until completely chilled.
9. Sprinkle 1 teaspoon of Swerve on top of each crème brûlée. Use the oven broiler to melt the sweetener.
10. Allow the topping to cool in the fridge for 5 minutes before serving.

Per Serving
calories: 138 | fat: 13.4g | protein: 2.0g | carbs: 2.3g | net carbs: 2.3g | fiber: 0g

Easy Flourless Chocolate Tortes

Prep time: 7 minutes | Cook time: 10 minutes | Serves 8

- ✿ 7 ounces (198 g) unsweetened baking chocolate, finely chopped
- ✿ ¾ cup plus 2 tablespoons unsalted butter (or butter-flavored coconut oil for dairy-free)
- ✿ 1¼ cups Swerve, or more to taste
- ✿ 5 large eggs
- ✿ 1 tablespoon coconut flour
- ✿ 2 teaspoons ground cinnamon
- ✿ Seeds scraped from 1 vanilla bean (about 8 inches long), or 2 teaspoons vanilla extract
- ✿ Pinch of fine sea salt

1. Grease 8 ramekins. Place the chocolate and butter in a pan over medium heat and stir until the chocolate is completely melted, about 3 minutes.
2. Remove the pan from the heat, then add the remaining ingredients and stir until smooth. Taste and adjust the sweetness to your liking. Pour the batter into the greased ramekins.
3. Place a trivet in the bottom of the Instant Pot and pour in 1 cup of cold water. Place four of the ramekins on the trivet.
4. Lock the lid. Select the Manual mode and set the cooking time for 7 minutes at High Pressure.
5. When the timer beeps, use a quick pressure release. Carefully remove the lid.
6. Use tongs to remove the ramekins. Repeat with the remaining ramekins.
7. Serve the tortes warm or chilled.

Per Serving
calories: 328 | fat: 27.5g | protein: 8.4g | carbs: 11.7g | net carbs: 7.2g | fiber: 4.5g

Chocolate Molten Cake

Prep time: 5 minutes | Cook time: 5 minutes | Serves 2

- ✿ 1 large egg
- ✿ 4 tablespoons unsweetened raw cocoa powder
- ✿ 2 tablespoons blanched almond flour
- ✿ 2 tablespoons Swerve
- ✿ 2 tablespoons full-fat heavy cream
- ✿ 1 teaspoon vanilla extract
- ✿ ½ teaspoon baking powder
- ✿ Pinch of sea salt
- ✿ 2 ounces (57 g) dark chocolate (at least 80% cacao), cut into chunks
- ✿ ½ cup water

1. In a small mixing bowl, beat the egg and add the cocoa powder, almond flour, Swerve, heavy cream, vanilla extract, baking powder and sea salt.
2. Transfer half of the batter into a small oven-proof bowl, add the dark chocolate pieces and then the rest of the batter. Loosely cover with aluminum foil.
3. Put the water in the Instant Pot and place the trivet inside. Place the bowl on the trivet.
4. Close the lid. Select on Manual mode and set the timer for 5 minutes on High pressure.
5. When timer beeps, use a natural pressure release for 5 minutes, then release any remaining pressure and open the lid.
6. Remove the bowl, uncover, and serve immediately.

Per Serving

calories: 287 | fat: 23.8g | protein: 17.2g | carbs: 8.0g | net carbs: 1.9g | fiber: 6.1g

Creamy Pine Nut Mousse

Prep time: 5 minutes | Cook time: 35 minutes | Serves 8

- ✿ 1 tablespoon butter
- ✿ 1¼ cups pine nuts
- ✿ 1¼ cups full-fat heavy cream
- ✿ 2 large eggs
- ✿ 1 teaspoon vanilla extract
- ✿ 1 cup Swerve, reserve 1 tablespoon
- ✿ 1 c water
- ✿ 1 cup full-fat heavy whipping cream

1. Butter the bottom and the side of a pie pan and set aside.
2. In a food processor, blend the pine nuts and heavy cream. Add the eggs, vanilla extract and Swerve and pulse a few times to incorporate.
3. Pour the batter into the pan and loosely cover with aluminum foil. Pour the water in the Instant Pot and place the trivet inside. Place the pan on top of the trivet.
4. Close the lid. Select Manual mode and set the timer for 35 minutes on High pressure.
5. In a small mixing bowl, whisk the heavy whipping cream and 1 tablespoon of Swerve until a soft peak forms.
6. When timer beeps, use a natural pressure release for 15 minutes, then release any remaining pressure and open the lid.
7. Serve immediately with whipped cream on top.

Per Serving

calories: 184 | fat: 18.8g | protein: 3.0g | carbs: 1.9g | net carbs: 1.8g | fiber: 0.1g

Lemon and Ricotta Torte

Prep time: 15 minutes | Cook time: 35 minutes | Serves 12

- ✿ Cooking spray

Torte:
- ✿ 1⅓ cups Swerve
- ✿ ½ cup (1 stick) unsalted butter, softened
- ✿ 2 teaspoons lemon or vanilla extract
- ✿ 5 large eggs, separated
- ✿ 2½ cups blanched almond flour

- ✿ 1¼ (10-ounce / 284-g) cups whole-milk ricotta cheese
- ✿ ¼ cup lemon juice
- ✿ 1 cup cold water

Lemon Glaze:
- ✿ ½ cup (1 stick) unsalted butter
- ✿ ¼ cup Swerve
- ✿ 2 tablespoons lemon juice

- ✿ 2 ounces (57 g) cream cheese (¼ cup)
- ✿ Grated lemon zest and lemon slices, for garnish

1. Line a baking pan with parchment paper and spray with cooking spray. Set aside.
2. Make the torte: In the bowl of a stand mixer, place the Swerve, butter, and extract and blend for 8 to 10 minutes until well combined. Scrape down the sides of the bowl as needed.
3. Add the egg yolks and continue to blend until fully combined. Add the almond flour and mix until smooth, then stir in the ricotta and lemon juice.
4. Whisk the egg whites in a separate medium bowl until stiff peaks form. Add the whites to the batter and stir well. Pour the batter into the prepared pan and smooth the top.
5. Place a trivet in the bottom of your Instant Pot and pour in the water. Use a foil sling to lower the baking pan onto the trivet. Tuck in the sides of the sling.
6. Seal the lid, press Pressure Cook or Manual, and set the timer for 30 minutes. Once finished, let the pressure release naturally.
7. Lock the lid. Select the Manual mode and set the cooking time for 30 minutes at High Pressure.
8. When the timer beeps, perform a natural pressure release for 10 minutes. Carefully remove the lid.
9. Use the foil sling to lift the pan out of the Instant Pot. Place the torte in the fridge for 40 minutes to chill before glazing.
10. Meanwhile, make the glaze: Place the butter in a large pan over high heat and cook for about 5 minutes until brown, stirring occasionally. Remove from the heat. While stirring the browned butter, add the Swerve.
11. Carefully add the lemon juice and cream cheese to the butter mixture. Allow the glaze to cool for a few minutes, or until it starts to thicken.
12. Transfer the chilled torte to a serving plate. Pour the glaze over the torte and return it to the fridge to chill for an additional 30 minutes.
13. Scatter the lemon zest on top of the torte and arrange the lemon slices on the plate around the torte.
14. Serve.

Per Serving
calories: 367 | fat: 32.8g | protein: 11.5g | carbs: 10.0g | net carbs: 7.0g | fiber: 3.0g

Deconstructed Tiramisu

Prep time: 5 minutes | Cook time: 9 minutes | Serves 4

- ✿ 1 cup heavy cream (or full-fat coconut milk for dairy-free)
- ✿ 2 large egg yolks
- ✿ 2 tablespoons brewed decaf espresso or strong brewed coffee
- ✿ 2 tablespoons Swerve, or more to taste
- ✿ 1 teaspoon rum extract
- ✿ 1 teaspoon unsweetened cocoa powder, or more to taste
- ✿ Pinch of fine sea salt
- ✿ 1 cup cold water
- ✿ 4 teaspoons Swerve, for topping

1. Heat the cream in a pan over medium-high heat until hot, about 2 minutes.
2. Place the egg yolks, coffee, sweetener, rum extract, cocoa powder, and salt in a blender and blend until smooth.
3. While the blender is running, slowly pour in the hot cream. Taste and adjust the sweetness to your liking. Add more cocoa powder, if desired.
4. Scoop the mixture into four ramekins with a spatula. Cover the ramekins with aluminum foil.
5. Place a trivet in the bottom of the Instant Pot and pour in the water. Place the ramekins on the trivet.
6. Lock the lid. Select the Manual mode and set the cooking time for 7 minutes at High Pressure.
7. When the timer beeps, use a quick pressure release. Carefully remove the lid.
8. Keep the ramekins covered with the foil and place in the refrigerator for about 2 hours until completely chilled.
9. Sprinkle 1 teaspoon of Swerve on top of each tiramisu. Use the oven broiler to melt the sweetener.
10. Put in the fridge to chill the topping, about 20 minutes.
11. Serve.

Per Serving
calories: 139 | fat: 13.4g | protein: 2.1g | carbs: 2.6g | net carbs: 2.5g | fiber: 0.1g

Grandma's Bread Pudding

Prep time: 5 minutes | Cook time: 10 minutes | Serves 18

- ✿ 1 Glazed Pumpkin Bundt Cake or Maple-Glazed Zucchini Bundt Cake, unglazed, cut into cubes (use zucchini cake for nut-free)
- ✿ 1 cup unsweetened almond milk (or full-fat coconut milk for nut-free)
- ✿ ½ cup heavy cream (or full-fat coconut milk for dairy-free)
- ✿ 3 large eggs
- ✿ ⅔ cup Swerve
- ✿ 1 teaspoon ground cinnamon
- ✿ Seeds scraped from 1 vanilla bean (about 8 inches long), or 2 teaspoons vanilla extract
- ✿ ½ teaspoon fine sea salt
- ✿ 1 cup cold water

Frosting:
- ✿ ½ cup unsalted butter (or butter-flavored coconut oil for dairy-free), softened
- ✿ ¼ cup Swerve, or more to taste
- ✿ 1 teaspoon ground cinnamon

1. In a large bowl, place the cake cubes and pour the milk and cream over them. Set aside.
2. Stir together the eggs, sweetener, cinnamon, and vanilla seeds in another large bowl. Pour the egg mixture over the soaked cake cubes and stir to combine.
3. Pour the cake mixture into a greased casserole dish.
4. Place a trivet in the bottom of the Instant Pot and pour in the water. Use a foil sling to lower the casserole dish onto the trivet. Tuck in the sides of the sling.
5. Lock the lid. Select the Manual mode and set the cooking time for 10 minutes at High Pressure.
6. When the timer beeps, use a natural pressure release for 10 minutes. Carefully remove the lid.
7. Use the foil sling to lift the dish out of the Instant Pot.
8. Allow the bread pudding to cool for 10 minutes before slicing.
9. Meanwhile, make the frosting: In a small bowl, stir in the softened butter, sweetener, and cinnamon. Taste and adjust the sweetness to your liking.
10. Serve warm or chilled. Dollop the frosting over the bread pudding slices.

Per Serving
calories: 367 | fat: 24.5g | protein: 4.1g | carbs: 30.4g | net carbs: 29.2g | fiber: 1.2g

Cinnamon Roll Cheesecake

Prep time: 15 minutes | Cook time: 35 minutes | Serves 12

Crust:
- 3½ tablespoons unsalted butter or coconut oil
- 1½ ounces (43 g) unsweetened baking chocolate, chopped
- 1 large egg, beaten
- ⅓ cup Swerve
- 2 teaspoons ground cinnamon
- 1 teaspoon vanilla extract
- ¼ teaspoon fine sea salt

Filling:
- 4 (8-ounce / 227-g) packages cream cheese, softened
- ¾ cup Swerve
- ½ cup unsweetened almond milk (or hemp milk for nut-free)
- 1 teaspoon vanilla extract
- ¼ teaspoon almond extract (omit for nut-free)
- ¼ teaspoon fine sea salt
- 3 large eggs

Cinnamon Swirl:
- 6 tablespoons (¾ stick) unsalted butter (or butter flavored coconut oil for dairy-free)
- ½ cup Swerve
- Seeds scraped from ½ vanilla bean (about 8 inches long), or 1 teaspoon vanilla
- extract
- 1 tablespoon ground cinnamon
- ¼ teaspoon fine sea salt
- 1 cup cold water

1. Line a baking pan with two layers of aluminum foil.
2. Make the crust: Melt the butter in a pan over medium-low heat. Slowly add the chocolate and stir until melted. Stir in the egg, sweetener, cinnamon, vanilla extract, and salt.
3. Transfer the crust mixture to the prepared baking pan, spreading it with your hands to cover the bottom completely.
4. Make the filling: In the bowl of a stand mixer, add the cream cheese, sweetener, milk, extracts, and salt and mix until well blended. Add the eggs, one at a time, mixing on low speed after each addition just until blended. Then blend until the filling is smooth. Pour half of the filling over the crust.
5. Make the cinnamon swirl: Heat the butter over high heat in a pan until the butter froths and brown flecks appear, stirring occasionally. Stir in the sweetener, vanilla seeds, cinnamon, and salt. Remove from the heat and allow to cool slightly.
6. Spoon half of the cinnamon swirl on top of the cheesecake filling in the baking pan. Use a knife to cut the cinnamon swirl through the filling several times for a marbled effect. Top with the rest of the cheesecake filling and cinnamon swirl. Cut the cinnamon swirl through the cheesecake filling again several times.
7. Place a trivet in the bottom of the Instant Pot and pour in the water. Use a foil sling to lower the baking pan onto the trivet. Cover the cheesecake with 3 large sheets of paper towel to ensure that condensation doesn't leak onto it. Tuck in the sides of the sling.
8. Lock the lid. Select the Manual mode and set the cooking time for 26 minutes at High Pressure.
9. When the timer beeps, use a natural pressure release for 10 minutes. Carefully remove the lid.
10. Use the foil sling to lift the pan out of the Instant Pot.
11. Let the cheesecake cool, then place in the refrigerator for 4 hours to chill and set completely before slicing and serving.

Per Serving
calories: 363 | fat: 34.2g | protein: 7.0g | carbs: 7.6g | net carbs: 6.4g | fiber: 1.2g

Glazed Pumpkin Bundt Cake

Prep time: 7 minutes | Cook time: 35 minutes | Serves 12

Cake:
- ✿ 3 cups blanched almond flour
- ✿ 1 teaspoon baking soda
- ✿ ½ teaspoon fine sea salt
- ✿ 2 teaspoons ground cinnamon
- ✿ 1 teaspoon ground nutmeg
- ✿ 1 teaspoon ginger powder
- ✿ ¼ teaspoon ground cloves
- ✿ 6 large eggs
- ✿ 2 cups pumpkin puree
- ✿ 1 cup Swerve
- ✿ ¼ cup (½ stick) unsalted butter (or coconut oil for dairy-free), softened

Glaze:
- ✿ 1 cup (2 sticks) unsalted butter (or coconut oil for dairy-free), melted
- ✿ ½ cup Swerve

1. In a large bowl, stir together the almond flour, baking soda, salt, and spices. In another large bowl, add the eggs, pumpkin, sweetener, and butter and stir until smooth. Pour the wet ingredients into the dry ingredients and stir well.
2. Grease a 6-cup Bundt pan. Pour the batter into the prepared pan and cover with a paper towel and then with aluminum foil.
3. Place a trivet in the bottom of the Instant Pot and pour in 2 cups of cold water. Place the Bundt pan on the trivet.
4. Lock the lid. Select the Manual mode and set the cooking time for 35 minutes at High Pressure.
5. When the timer beeps, use a natural pressure release for 10 minutes. Carefully remove the lid.
6. Let the cake cool in the pot for 10 minutes before removing.
7. While the cake is cooling, make the glaze: In a small bowl, mix the butter and sweetener together. Spoon the glaze over the warm cake.
8. Allow to cool for 5 minutes before slicing and serving.

Per Serving
calories: 332 | fat: 21.9g | protein: 6.8g | carbs: 27.4g | net carbs: 26.2g | fiber: 1.2g

Mini Maple Bacon Upside-Down Cheesecakes

Prep time: 15 minutes | Cook time: 10 minutes | Serves 8

- ✿ 3 (8-ounce/ 227-g) packages cream cheese, softened
- ✿ ⅔ cup Swerve
- ✿ ½ cup unsweetened almond milk (or hemp milk for nut-free)
- ✿ 2 teaspoons maple extract
- ✿ ¼ teaspoon fine sea salt
- ✿ 1 large egg
- ✿ 4 slices bacon, chopped, for topping
- ✿ Sweetened Whipped Cream:
- ✿ ½ cup heavy cream
- ✿ 2 tablespoons Swerve, or more to taste

1. In the bowl of a stand mixer, add the cream cheese, sweetener, milk, maple extract, and salt and blitz until well blended. Add the egg and mix on low speed until very smooth.
2. Pour the batter into 8 ramekins. Gently tap the ramekins against the counter to bring the air bubbles to the surface.
3. Place a trivet in the bottom of the Instant Pot and pour in 1 cup of cold water. Stack the ramekins in two layers on top of the trivet. Cover the top layer of ramekins with 3 large pieces of paper towel to ensure that condensation doesn't leak onto the cheesecakes.
4. Lock the lid. Select the Manual mode and set the cooking time for 6 minutes at High Pressure.
5. When the timer beeps, use a natural pressure release for 10 minutes. Carefully remove the lid.
6. Remove the ramekins with tongs.
7. Place the cheesecakes in the fridge to chill completely, about 4 hours.
8. Meanwhile, make the topping: Cook the bacon in a skillet over medium-high heat for 4 minutes until crisp and cooked through. Place the cooked bacon on a paper towel–lined plate to drain.
9. Add the cream to a medium bowl and use a hand mixer on high speed to mix until soft peaks form. Fold in the sweetener and mix until well combined. Taste and adjust the sweetness to your liking.
10. Drizzle with the sweetened whipped cream and place the bacon on top.
11. Serve.

Per Serving
calories: 371 | fat: 34.4g | protein: 8.7g | carbs: 8.0g | net carbs: 7.9g | fiber: 0.1g

Maple-Glazed Zucchini Bundt Cake

Prep time: 7 minutes | Cook time: 40 minutes | Serves 8

Cake:

- ✿ 6 large eggs
- ✿ 1 cup full-fat coconut milk
- ✿ ¾ cup (1½ sticks) unsalted butter (or butter-flavored coconut oil for dairy-free), melted
- ✿ ½ cup Swerve

- ✿ 2 teaspoons ground cinnamon
- ✿ 1 cup coconut flour
- ✿ 1 teaspoon fine sea salt
- ✿ 1 teaspoon baking powder
- ✿ 1 cup shredded zucchini
- ✿ 3 teaspoons vanilla extract

Maple Glaze:

- ✿ ½ cup (1 stick) unsalted butter (or butter-flavored coconut oil for dairy-free)
- ✿ ¼ cup Swerve
- ✿ 2 ounces (57 g) cream cheese (¼ cup) (or

Kite Hill brand cream cheese style spread for dairy-free)
- ✿ Chopped raw walnuts, for garnish (omit for nut-free)

1. Whisk the eggs with a hand mixer until light and foamy in large bowl. Stir in the coconut milk, melted butter, sweetener, and cinnamon.
2. In another large bowl, stir together the coconut flour, salt, and baking powder. Add the dry ingredients to the wet ingredients and stir well, then fold in the shredded zucchini and extract and stir again.
3. Grease a 6-cup Bundt pan. Pour the batter into the prepared pan and cover the pan with a paper towel and then with aluminum foil.
4. Place a trivet in the bottom of the Instant Pot and pour in 2 cups of cold water. Place the Bundt pan on the trivet.
5. Lock the lid. Select the Manual mode and set the cooking time for 35 minutes at High Pressure.
6. When the timer beeps, use a natural pressure release for 10 minutes. Carefully remove the lid.
7. Let the cake cool in the pot for 10 minutes before removing.
8. Chill the cake in the fridge or freezer before removing from the Bundt pan, about 1 hour.
9. While the cake is cooling, make the glaze: Place the butter in a large pan over high heat and cook for about 5 minutes until brown, stirring occasionally.
10. Remove from the heat. While stirring the browned butter, vigorously, add the sweetener.
11. Carefully add the cream cheese and maple extract to the butter mixture. Allow the glaze to cool for a few minutes, or until it starts to thicken.
12. Transfer the chilled cake to a serving plate and drizzle the glaze over the top. Sprinkle with the walnuts while the glaze is still wet.
13. Place the cake in the fridge to chill completely for an additional 30 minutes before serving.

Per Serving
calories: 378 | fat: 30.1g | protein: 9.8g | carbs: 17.4g | net carbs: 15.9g | fiber: 1.5g

Espresso Cheesecake with Raspberries

Prep time: 5 minutes | Cook time: 35 minutes | Serves 8

- ✿ 1 cup blanched almond flour
- ✿ ½ cup plus 2 tablespoons Swerve
- ✿ 3 tablespoons espresso powder, divided
- ✿ 2 tablespoons butter
- ✿ 1 egg
- ✿ ½ cup full-fat heavy cream
- ✿ 16 ounces (454 g) cream cheese
- ✿ 1 cup water
- ✿ 6 ounces (170 g) dark chocolate (at least 80% cacao)
- ✿ 8 ounces (227 g) full-fat heavy whipping cream
- ✿ 2 cups raspberries

1. In a small mixing bowl, combine the almond flour, 2 tablespoons of Swerve, 1 tablespoon of espresso powder and the butter.
2. Line the bottom of a springform pan with parchment paper. Press the almond flour dough flat on the bottom and about 1 inch on the sides. Set aside.
3. In a food processor, mix the egg, heavy cream, cream cheese, remaining Swerve and remaining espresso powder until smooth.
4. Pour the cream cheese mixture into the springform pan. Loosely cover with aluminum foil.
5. Put the water in the Instant Pot and place the trivet inside.
6. Close the lid. Select Manual button and set the timer for 35 minutes on High pressure.
7. When timer beeps, use a natural pressure release for 15 minutes, then release any remaining pressure. Open the lid.
8. Remove the springform pan and place it on a cooling rack for 2 to 3 hours or until it reaches room temperature. Refrigerate overnight.
9. Melt the chocolate and heavy whipping cream in the double boiler. Cool for 15 minutes and drizzle on top of the cheesecake, allowing the chocolate to drip down the sides.
10. Add the raspberries on top of the cheesecake before serving.

Per Serving
calories: 585 | fat: 53.8g | protein: 12.2g | carbs: 14.9g | net carbs: 10.8g | fiber: 4.1g

Appendix 1: 28-Day Keto Meal Plan

	Breakfast	Lunch	Dinner
1	Classic Cinnamon Roll Coffee Cake	Beef Back Ribs with Barbecue Glaze	Stir-Fry Shrimp and Cauliflower
2	Gruyère Asparagus Frittata	Lime Cauliflower Rice with Cilantro	Albóndigas Sinaloenses
3	Streusel Pumpkin Cake	Herb and Lemon Whole Chicken	Beef Brisket with Cabbage
4	Sumptuous Breakfast Stuffed Mushrooms	Broccoli and Bacon Cheese Soup	Bacon-Wrapped Pork Bites
5	Bacon and Mushroom Quiche Lorraine	Beef Carne Guisada	Cheesy Trout Casserole
6	Warm Breakfast Salad with Sardines	Barbecue Shredded Chicken	Spaghetti Squash Noodles with Tomatoes
7	Peppery Ham Frittata	Beef Cheeseburger Pie	Chicken Escabèche
8	Bacon and Spinach Eggs	Aromatic Pork Steak Curry	Garlic Tuna Casserole
9	Sumptuous Breakfast Stuffed Mushrooms	Lemony Asparagus with Gremolata	Mexican Chicken and Avocado Soup
10	Broccoli, Ham, and Pepper Frittata	Cheesy Chicken Casserole	Garlicky Broccoli with Roasted Almonds
11	Easy Eggs Benedict	Beef Masala Curry	Beery Boston-Style Butt
12	Almond Butter Beef Bowl	Broiled Cauli Bites	Thai Coconut Chicken
13	Pumpkin Cake with Walnuts	Spicy Shrimp Salad	Rainbow Trout with Mixed Greens
14	Flavor-Packed Breakfast Pizza	Halibut Stew with Bacon and Cheese	Hearty Chuck Roast and Vegetable Stew

15	Gruyère Asparagus Frittata	Tuna Salad with Tomatoes and Peppers	Beef Ribs with Radishes
16	Bacon and Mushroom Quiche Lorraine	Beef Shawarma and Veggie Salad Bowls	Green Garden Soup
17	Kale and Sausage Egg Muffins	Classic Osso Buco with Gremolata	Avocado and Serrano Chile Soup
18	Streusel Pumpkin Cake	Beef and Okra Stew	Easy Pork Steaks with Pico de Gallo
19	Peppery Ham Frittata	Garlicky Buttery Whole Cauliflower	BLT Chicken Salad
20	Broccoli, Ham, and Pepper Frittata	Beef Shoulder Roast	Chicken and Scallions Stuffed Peppers
21	Almond Butter Beef Bowl	Blue Cheese Mushroom Soup	Harissa Lamb
22	Chorizo and Egg Lettuce Tacos	Lemony Fish and Asparagus	Baked Cheesy Mushroom Chicken
23	Classic Cinnamon Roll Coffee Cake	Falafel and Lettuce Salad	Cauliflower Rice and Chicken Thigh Soup
24	Pumpkin Cake with Walnuts	Satarash with Eggs	Swai with Port Wine Sauce
25	Streusel Pumpkin Cake	Cheesy Pesto Chicken	Eggplant Pork Lasagna
26	Bacon and Broccoli Frittata	Cheesy Bacon Stuffed Meatloaf	Garam Masala Fish
27	Flavor-Packed Breakfast Pizza	Beef Meatball Minestrone	Italian Sausage Stuffed Bell Peppers
28	Warm Breakfast Salad with Sardines	Beef, Bacon and Cauliflower Rice Casserole	Baked Cheesy Mushroom Chicken

Appendix 2: Measurement Conversion Chart

VOLUME EQUIVALENTS(DRY)

US STANDARD	METRIC (APPROXIMATE)
1/8 teaspoon	0.5 mL
1/4 teaspoon	1 mL
1/2 teaspoon	2 mL
3/4 teaspoon	4 mL
1 teaspoon	5 mL
1 tablespoon	15 mL
1/4 cup	59 mL
1/2 cup	118 mL
3/4 cup	177 mL
1 cup	235 mL
2 cups	475 mL
3 cups	700 mL
4 cups	1 L

VOLUME EQUIVALENTS(LIQUID)

US STANDARD	US STANDARD (OUNCES)	METRIC (APPROXIMATE)
2 tablespoons	1 fl.oz.	30 mL
1/4 cup	2 fl.oz.	60 mL
1/2 cup	4 fl.oz.	120 mL
1 cup	8 fl.oz.	240 mL
1 1/2 cup	12 fl.oz.	355 mL
2 cups or 1 pint	16 fl.oz.	475 mL
4 cups or 1 quart	32 fl.oz.	1 L
1 gallon	128 fl.oz.	4 L

TEMPERATURES EQUIVALENTS

FAHRENHEIT(F)	CELSIUS(C) (APPROXIMATE)
225 °F	107 °C
250 °F	120 °C
275 °F	135 °C
300 °F	150 °C
325 °F	160 °C
350 °F	180 °C
375 °F	190 °C
400 °F	205 °C
425 °F	220 °C
450 °F	235 °C
475 °F	245 °C
500 °F	260 °C

WEIGHT EQUIVALENTS

US STANDARD	METRIC (APPROXIMATE)
1 ounce	28 g
2 ounces	57 g
5 ounces	142 g
10 ounces	284 g
15 ounces	425 g
16 ounces (1 pound)	455 g
1.5 pounds	680 g
2 pounds	907 g

Appendix 3: References

Centers for Disease Control and Prevention. (2020). National diabetes statistics report 2020: Estimates of diabetes and its burden in the United States. https://www.cdc.gov/diabetes/pdfs/data/statistics/national-diabetes-statistics-report.pdf

Figure 1: Katherine Chase. (2018). Gray and black rice cooker [Photograph]. Unsplash. https://unsplash.com/photos/VNBUJ6imfGs

Figure 2: Eduardo Roda Lopes. (2017). Person holding white ceramic plate [Photograph]. Unsplash. https://unsplash.com/photos/mNefYU7uRbk

Figure 3: Nadine Primeau. (2019). Sliced broccoli and cucumber on a plate with grey stainless steel fork near bell pepper, snow peas, avocado fruit [Photograph]. Unsplash. https://unsplash.com/photos/l5MjI9qH8VU

Figure 4: Alex Munsell. (2015). Close-up photo of cooked food on white square plate [Photograph]. Unsplash. https://unsplash.com/photos/auIbTAcSH6E

Kroemer, G., Lopez-Otin, C., Madeo, F. & Cabo, R. (2018). Carbotoxicity: Noxious effects of carbohydrates. Cell, 175(3), 605-614. https://www.sciencedirect.com/science/article/pii/S0092867418309723

Manikam, N., Pantoro, N., Komala, K. & Sari, A. (2018). Comparing the efficacy of ketogenic diet with low-fat diet for weight loss in obesity Patients: Evidence-based case report. Research Gate. https://www.researchgate.net/publication/327189134_Comparing_the_Efficacy_of_Ketogenic_Diet_with_Low-Fat_Diet_for_Weight_Loss_in_Obesity_Patients_Evidenc-Based_Case_Report

Masood, W., Annamaraju, P. & Uppulari, K.R. (2020). Ketogenic diet. NCBI. https://www.ncbi.nlm.nih.gov/books/NBK499830/

Nam, K.H., Yeong An, S., Su Joo, Y., Lee, S., Yun, H., Jhee, J.H., Han, S.H., Yoo, T.H., Kang, S. & Park, J.T. (2019). Carbohydrate-rich diet is associated with increased risk of incident chronic kidney disease in non-diabetic subjects. U.S. National Library of Medicine National Institute of Health. https://www.ncbi.nlm.nih.gov/pmc/articles/PMC6617052/

Robert, S.B. (2000). High-glycemic index foods, hunger, and obesity: Is there a connection? PubMed. https://pubmed.ncbi.nlm.nih.gov/10885323/

Westman, E.C., Yancy, W.S., Mavropoulos, J.C., Marquart, M. & McDuffie, J.R. (2008). The effect of a low-carbohydrate, ketogenic diet versus a low-glycemic index diet on glycemic control in type 2 diabetes mellitus. U.S. National Library of Medicine National Institute of Health. https://www.ncbi.nlm.nih.gov/pmc/articles/PMC2633336/

Printed by Amazon Italia Logistica S.r.l.
Torrazza Piemonte (TO), Italy